Powerlifting

Training, Techniques and Performance

Nicola Vaughan-Ellis

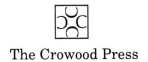

The Crowood Press

First published in 2013 by
The Crowood Press Ltd
Ramsbury, Marlborough
Wiltshire SN8 2HR

www.crowood.com

British Library Cataloguing-in-Publication Data
A catalogue record for this book is available from the British Library.

ISBN 978 1 84797 574 4

Project editor: Margo Galvin
Photographs of the three powerlifting lifts © Terry Galvin
Anatomical drawings © Caryl Dane
All other photographs © Nicola Vaughan-Ellis and Margo Galvin

Typeset by Jean Cussons Typesetting, Diss, Norfolk
Printed and bound in India by Replika Press Pvt Ltd

CONTENTS

DEDICATION

To my granddaughter, Tabitha, the first of a new generation. She is symbolic of the possibilities of altering the orientations of the time and space we occupy. May it be a positive journey.

'In all things, success depends on previous preparation, and without such preparation there is sure to be failure.'

Confucius (c55–c478BC)

ACKNOWLEDGEMENTS

The following unique group of individuals has been extremely helpful in making this book possible: Margo Galvin, my ever-patient editor; illustrator Caryl Dane and photographer Terry Galvin. My sincere thanks go to all three for their exceptional expertise and valuable time. My gratitude also goes to all of the coaches and service providers that I have met during my career. All of the above have been indispensible to my vision of bringing Powerlifting to a general readership.

FOREWORD

With an ever-escalating interest in sport and the national heroes of the London 2012 Olympics and Paralympics Games, it is not hard to notice the growing number of books being published on such themes as the Olympic experience and what it takes to become an elite athlete or world-class coach. Many of these books are academic in nature, examining the regimes, skills and advanced techniques that have enabled athletes to train their minds and bodies in order to become the best. Other titles are autobiographies by top athletes describing their experiences at world class level. Very few marry the two aspects together and even fewer achieve this for the sport of powerlifting.

In *Powerlifting: Skills, Training and Techniques* Nicola Vaughan-Ellis sets out to bridge this gap and, in my view, succeeds admirably. This is not just another strength training book. Certainly, it contains comprehensive examples of training programmes that the author has developed over thirty years. However, it extends well beyond this to include technical explanations and illustrations of the three powerlifting lifts, detailed discussion of the role of the coach enriched with her own coaching philosophy and a step-by-step breakdown of what happens at a powerlifting competition.

What sets this book apart from other titles is its fusion of academic insight and real life experience gained at the highest level, all brought to life with authentic sporting examples and practical tips that the reader can easily follow. Underpinning it all is Ms Vaughan-Ellis' passion for the sport of powerlifting and for the emerging generation of coaches and athletes who are carrying the sport forward.

I met Ms Vaughan-Ellis when I became her mentor in 2006 while she was preparing for her coaching role at the Beijing Paralympics Games (her third Games). Since then, I have watched her progress and witnessed at first-hand her passion, dedication and drive to develop the sport of powerlifting. She has gained global recognition and respect as an athlete, coach, referee and manager while striving to create a climate of excellence that is enriched by deep knowledge and leading-edge ideas. All of this, I believe, makes her ideally placed to examine and explain how the coach, athlete and the athlete's wider support network work together to grow and succeed within the sport.

The challenge for the author is to present an interesting, useful and reader-friendly text. Even though powerlifting is not my primary sport, my attention was captured and my interest sustained as I reviewed the various topics in this book. Ms Vaughan-Ellis has an instinct for what is right and what will work, and translates this into practical steps, supported by real life examples, that the athlete can take to improve their performance and achieve – even exceed – their powerlifting goals.

I was particularly impressed by the clear explanation of the different stages of skill and technical development required to perform the three powerlifting lifts and the strategies available to help the athlete put the theory into practice. The writing style is clear and the contents are presented in an interesting and thought-provoking manner. Feature boxes and clear photographs and diagrams help to illustrate key points throughout the book.

Ms Vaughan-Ellis does not attempt to include

every topic or theme associated with powerlifting and the complementary sciences relating to the elite athlete. I believe this is a wise decision as it is quite impossible to do justice to all topics involved. She has focused on what is involved in developing the skills and techniques required to become an accomplished powerlifter and how the coach, athlete and supporting service providers work together to achieve the desired outcomes. While there is much in this book for the afore-mentioned individuals, the powerlifting enthusiast and the general lover of sport should also find plenty to enjoy.

Ms Vaughan-Ellis has produced a long awaited book of substance for the sport of powerlifting. Importantly, I believe it clearly illustrates how and why powerlifting has earned its place at the highest level of international competition, placing it alongside other world ranking strength sports. This is an informative, enjoyable read and I welcome its addition to the growing catalogue of sporting titles.

Peter A. Hirst

Former Performance and Coaching Director of England Squash, and former head of Coaching New Zealand.

INTRODUCTION

This book is a guide to athletes and coaches in powerlifting, as well as a more general book for sports lovers. It takes a coach-led, athlete-centred approach that is intended to empower the individual, promote excellence and facilitate personal fulfilment within the sport.

Powerlifting is fundamentally a sport that requires the athlete to pit themselves against the weight to be lifted, but it is important to remember that this cannot be achieved by the individual alone. It requires teamwork, support, and the sharing of knowledge, ideas and honest and constructive feedback. Therefore, in this book, I have described the preparation required by the individual athlete to perform each lift safely and successfully, as well as the skills required by the athlete's coach and support network in helping them along their chosen pathway.

There are many books available that cover specific aspects of training, from training programmes (what is prescriptive) and training cycles (the activities the body goes through to complete the programme) to loading, strength building and adaptation of the mind and body, to name a few. All of these are excellent individual training components.

However, this book takes a different approach in that it offers a fusion of many different ideas in an easy-to-apply framework. It takes a multi-faceted, holistic and yet fluid view, based on the belief that 'the sum of the whole' will provide a well grounded formula that is close to the needs of the athlete. It combines the scientific and statistical elements that underpin training loads with the physical and artistic elements that enable the athlete to create the optimal body shape to facilitate the correct pathway of the lifting bar. Above all, this book reflects my belief that the key to any successful training programme is not the 'what' but the 'how'.

The book is divided into three sections which can be read in isolation or consecutively. Part 1 examines and unpicks the three powerlifting lifts of the squat, bench press and deadlift, analyzing the skills and techniques required to perform each lift successfully within the context of good practice. It also discusses the Paralympic bench press for athletes with a disability, as it is an integral part of the sport today. Part 2 looks at the role of the coach, describing the coaching pathway within a powerlifting context and providing guidelines that will help the coach help their athlete/s achieve their desired process goals and performance targets. In Part 3 the focus shifts to competition and all that it entails, including the role of the coach in deciding competition strategy and the responsibilities of the athlete, in particular in relation to drug testing.

There are various powerlifting federations within the UK and around the world. This book primarily identifies with the Great Britain Powerlifting Federation (GBPF), the powerlifting arm of the International Paralympic Committee (IPC) and British Weight Lifting (BWL). These bodies are recognized by UK Sport and Sport England and adhere to the World Anti-Doping Federation (WADA). They also provide coaching courses, athlete education and athlete performance pathways.

Whether athlete or coach, the reader of this book should come away with an improved understanding of the three powerlifting lifts and valuable insights into preparing for and delivering a successful competition performance.

PART I

THE LIFTS

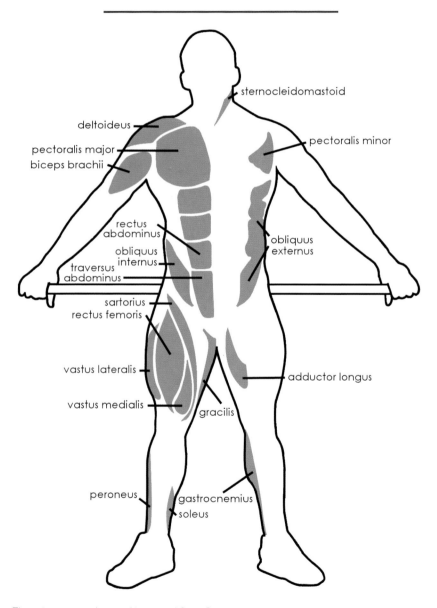

sternocleidomastoid

deltoideus

pectoralis minor

pectoralis major

biceps brachii

rectus
abdominus

obliquus
externus

obliquus
internus

traversus
abdominus

sartorius

rectus femoris

vastus lateralis

adductor longus

vastus medialis

gracilis

peroneus

gastrocnemius

soleus

The primary muscles used in powerlifting, front view.

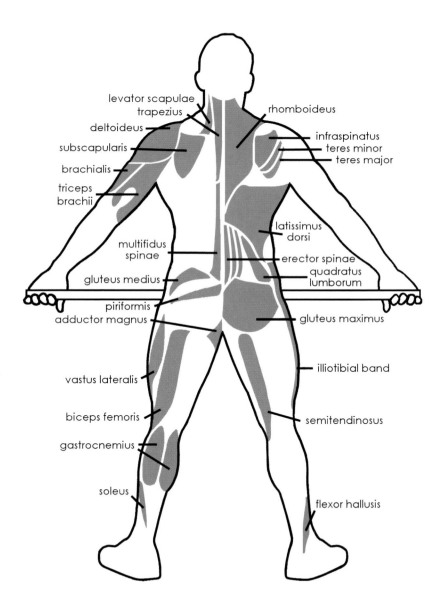

levator scapulae
trapezius
deltoideus
subscapularis
brachialis
triceps
brachii
multifidus
spinae
gluteus medius
piriformis
adductor magnus
vastus lateralis
biceps femoris
gastrocnemius
soleus

rhomboideus
infraspinatus
teres minor
teres major
latissimus
dorsi
erector spinae
quadratus
lumborum
gluteus maximus
illiotibial band
semitendinosus
flexor hallusis

The primary muscles used in powerlifting, back view.

CHAPTER 1

THE SQUAT

The squat is known as the king of the strength exercises, as world class lifters can squat weights in excess of three times their body weight. The lift predominantly utilizes the legs, back and a well-developed core. Consequently, the best squatters are known for having extremely well developed quadriceps and latissimus dorsi muscles, although it should be noted that the squat is an excellent exercise for the whole body.

Indeed, squatting with correct technique following a well-designed progressive training programme is known to promote collagen activity, improve bone density, assist hypertrophy and help improve body posture and flexibility while challenging the lifter's mental aptitude. It offers additional potential benefits to female lifters since, as well as promoting bone density, it is associated with the possible delay of osteoporosis. Moreover, athletes who use the squat via progressive loading phases as a mainstay of their exercise regime appear to be less vulnerable to fractures.

The squat is the first lift in a powerlifting competition and is considered to be the ultimate test of strength and power for the majority of athletes who lift weights. Top squatters are naturally inclined towards training their legs and have a genetic propensity for a strong lumbar (mid to lower) region of the back. However, they are also prepared to train their core as intensively as their back and legs. They often have a shorter lumbar region and shorter levers (such as the femur) which may have huge muscle bulk attached together with good flexibility in the shoulders, hips and ankles. Good squatters must be able to fight against gravity with all of their muscle groups, since during the lift the lifting bar is forced down and forward, potentially causing the athlete to fold in half or lose their balance.

There are different styles of squat, with each having its own training and competition criteria. For bodybuilders the aim may be to promote hypertrophy (increased muscle size), in which case they will favour the back squat. Competitive weightlifters may want to strengthen another lift, for example increase the 'clean' in the clean and jerk, and they will favour the front squat. Alternatively, the squat may be the prime focus and test of power and strength for a competitive powerlifter, who will only use the back squat in competition.

A powerlifting back squat differs from the bodybuilding back squat in that, as stated above, the aim of the latter is to promote muscle growth and density. As such, the bodybuilder will train the back squat with more repetitions (between fifteen and twenty in any given training session) than both the powerlifter (who would generally do no more than eight) and the weightlifter (who would use it as a secondary exercise). In addition, unlike the powerlifter, the bodybuilder will not usually break parallel (bring the hips below the knees) during the lift, and in order to perform the lift they will adopt a stance and 'frame' that is different from that of the powerlifter.

An International Powerlifting Federation (IPF) back squat, performed in both equipped and unequipped competitions, requires a lifter to lift a maximum load safely as a test of strength and power. To verify this strength there are rules written around the lift which apply from the moment the lifter stands erect with the weight to the point where they make a *bona fide* attempt to return the weight to the designated safety racks. The lift commences with the loaded bar being placed across the lifter's upper back. The lifter then steps away from the safety racks, squats to below parallel (with the hips below the knees) and pushes back up again for one repetition, with the whole process being validated by designated referees. It should be noted here that in some competitions, as is often the case in the US, the interpretation of breaking parallel differs and as a result the lifter's hips may be more in line with the knee. Regardless of the powerlifting federations' differing criteria, however, the organizations all subscribe to the view that the most weight lifted compared to body weight and ratified in competition is the result of the powerlifting back squat.

While each of the three types of squat is employed for different outcomes and produces a slightly different emphasis on how the leg muscles grow and become defined, they all share some commonalities. For example, each lift requires a strong lower back and the ability to hold the bar in place with the chosen grip for the duration of the lift as well as the confidence to get under heavy tonnage, control the weight from an elected start position, squat down with the weight under control and stand back up again.

Performing the Squat

The lifter places their hands on the loaded bar, allowing enough space to move their torso

TRAINED LOADERS

In order to lift heavy weights safely it is wise to engage the help of trained loaders. These are individuals who understand the biomechanics of the three powerlifting lifts, how to load the bar and when to intervene if a lifter is likely to fail the lift or lose control of the weight.

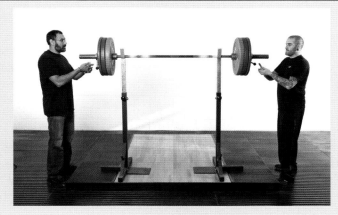

Above: Initial position of loaders for the squat.

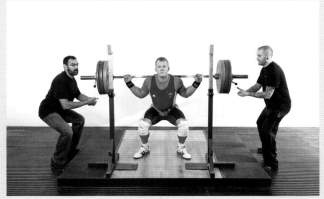

Left: Loaders shadowing the lifter as they perform the exercise.

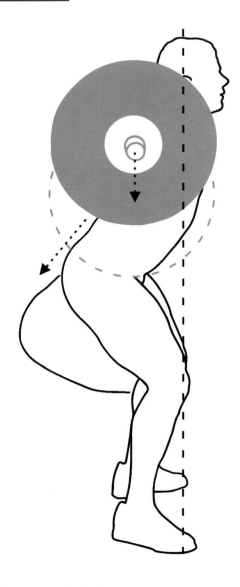

Quarter squat, body alignment.

point, since they will be lifting the loaded bar as well as a proportion of their own body weight.

When the lifter has positioned the bar comfortably across their shoulders, they should stand upright, clear the weighted bar from the safety racks and step out of the power racks. To do this they should move one leg backwards and to the side, adopting a suitable stance. When the foot is firmly placed on the floor the second foot should follow and move to the opposite side. This manoeuvre takes time to practise, as the lifter needs to move into their lifting stance smoothly and swiftly without causing the body to take the entire load at an angle that it is not designed to do. Stepping out at this point with the bar twisting under the weight may cause injury.

Once the lifter has found their elected stance, moved clear of the safety racks and is standing upright with chest up and out they must not allow the weight of the bar to push them forward by more than 15 degrees from what the referees consider to be the lifter's upright position. When their knees are locked and the bar is no more than 3cm below the deltoid (see federation rules) the referee will grant them the start signal.

At the start of the descent phase the feet must be flat on the floor, with the knees not pushing forward past the toes behind them, as the hips draw backwards and down. The back should remain as upright as possible. The knees begin to move apart, with the feet remaining flat and in contact with the ground and the ankles flexing so that the weight is kept behind the knees as they continue to widen; the back is kept tight and upright. This forges a gap for the hips to slide through as the torso descends. It is here that the shoulders and back are most likely to tip too far forward. This can force the head to fall forward, stopping the hips from descending further and often preventing the lifter from breaking parallel. This is a common failure for the squat discipline under IPF rules.

When the lifter has reached the bottom of the descent they must then push up through the feet

through the space between their hands. They then step under the bar, with head and knees bent and subscapularis (shoulder blades) pulled together, and finally position their feet directly below it. The lifter must then begin to push up slightly against the bar and nestle the trapezius muscles under it. It is imperative that the lifter creates a stable base from which to squat at this

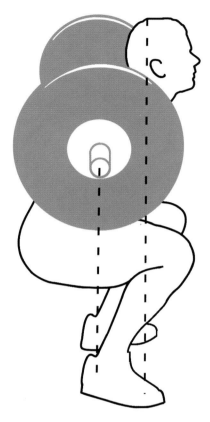

Parallel squat, hip to knee and knee to ankle alignment (note: this is not below parallel).

and trapezius muscles. This is achieved by leading with the chest and pushing up through the sternum, keeping the scapulae pulled together and holding the knees wide until the hips have just begun to push back and through to neutral. The knees should then be pulled back in line with the ankles as the lifter ascends. The lifter should keep moving forward and up, resisting the pressure to push too far forward and allow the weight to transcend from the lower part of the body to the upper and over the toes. As the lifter passes three quarters of the way through the lift they must try to pull up and back, keeping the weight over the heels. Once upright, the lifter should lock the knees and stand still while awaiting the chief referee's signal to rack the bar.

Once the signal is granted the lifter must make a valid attempt to walk the bar back into the racks. To do this they should walk forward one step at a time, bending the head, lowering the shoulders and slightly bending the knees again to place the bar back in the squat racks. The spotters are permitted to assist once the final signal has been given by the chief referee.

Anatomy

Skeletal system
The skeletal system is the framework of bones that forms the base and shape for muscles and tendons to attach to. This framework dictates an individual lifter's biomechanical levers which in turn influence the lifting technique that should be adopted. The density, length, symmetry and any previous breaks in bones will influence the type of exercises selected for the lifter's training programme.

Back
In the squat, the spine is the long lever arm of the fulcrum. It must maintain shape and form throughout – that is at least a 45 degree angle – and should not be allowed to bend (fold). The lower lumbar region can hyper-extend slightly to control the axis as the lifter descends and ascends.

Novices or lifters who have not received good coaching often drop too quickly on the descent of the squat, with little control. This can place too much pressure on the lower back and lead to injury. Another common fault which has dramatic effects on the lower back is when the lifter folds in the middle, losing control of the weight and their shoulders moving forward over the knees.

Back problems are usually attributed to squatting, with the majority of cases caused by poor technique. A lifter may train with poor technique for a few months, even years, if they have very strong muscle groups. However, as the nature of lifting is to lift progressively heavier and heavier weights, lifters often move on to the next stage before they have fully mastered the more complex body position required at this level, thus risking injury.

Alternatively, a lifter may increase the weight before all the appropriate muscle groups are capable of taking the extra load. For example, a lifter with very strong legs and lower back but little flexibility in the shoulder joints due to over-tight pectoral muscles, and with slightly weaker rear deltoids, will round their shoulders too much under load, putting added strain on the middle back and resulting in extra forward movement. The legs will keep strong and hold form and therefore the body will continue to go up and down in the squat exercise. However, the lifter will not realize they are becoming more and more bent over during the ascent phase of the lift. Eventually they will assume some break in form is normal due to the weight being so heavy. However, the reality will be that a fundamental element of their technique has broken down. This leads to displacement of the centre of gravity which can in turn pull the pelvic muscles, sacrum and connecting erector, causing soft tissue damage or spinal misalignment and disc compression.

Finally, if the lifter squats with the bar close to the base of the neck and tips forward, the bar can easily roll up the neck. The lifter may then lose control of the bar which could roll over the head, potentially causing lifelong damage or, in extreme cases, fatality.

Hips

The hips are integral to the squat (as the elbows are in the bench press) since they, and the muscles linked with the pelvis, promote movement in the legs. Most strength-based athletes train their squat in one particular line for years. This is fine for perfecting a particular movement for competition and building strength to promote hypertrophy. However, it does mean that the majority of lifters develop an imbalance in the alignment of the pelvis and hips. If the whole area is not trained, poor technique will result since the route for power to be transmitted from the legs to the upper body will be hindered, forcing an unnecessary load onto the hips and pelvis. This can leave lifters with tight hip flexors and restricted movement when performing their adopted squat, eventually building a route for injury to set in.

Knees

When squatting, the lifter's knees must be positioned behind the toes to avoid the risk of knee injury and on the ascent should be pushed wide with the shins remaining vertical. A below parallel squat will take some pressure off the knees by transferring the load to the hips. Also, if the legs are strong enough to warrant a wider stance, this will reduce knee torque – where all of the forces of gravity focus on one place.

The knees become vulnerable if the lifter is significantly weaker in the calves compared to the upper legs. The main risk occurs if the calves and hamstrings bounce off one another at the bottom of the squat. This occurs if the lifter does not control the downward phase, for example by dropping down too quickly with little control in the movement, as this forces the knees to act like breaks, a task they are not designed for, which can cause a dislocation effect.

Knee injuries are commonly associated with squatting, with most injuries caused by an imbalance in muscle maturity and a lack of flexibility. For example, very tight hip flexors can stop the lifter drawing their hips back far enough at the beginning of the descent of the lift. Therefore, as the lifter continues to descend with the weight, the restricted movement causes the knees to slide forward over the toes and take strain they were not designed for.

Abdominals

The abdominals bridge the gap between the pelvis and the thorax and play an important role in all three powerlifting lifts. If there is an imbalance between the abdominals and the development of the back this can cause a lifter to fold under the squat, resulting in too much pressure being placed on the back. When squatters complain of back pain this is often due to having a weak abdominal wall, and this in turn makes the spine more prone to injury.

Within the world of powerlifting there is no denying that the abdominals support the trunk when executing the three lifts. Nevertheless, there are different schools of thought about how and when to train abdominals. Some would say that by training the three lifts, this is enough to tighten and strengthen the abdominals for the movements needed. Others believe that as the lifter advances they should undertake a core programme that can be done daily outside their strength training.

Either way, if the body is to become a tool capable of moving large tonnage there is a huge disadvantage to having a steel-like back and an abdomen akin to soft cotton wool balls. Hence, a well-developed core will help the body to distribute the load when dealing with such heavy tonnage.

THE SQUAT MOVEMENT

According to the lifter's technique the order of muscle firing may vary slightly, but the following would be a typical movement.

Taking the weight from the racks

- Select the preferred grip.
- Dip under the bar.
- Pin shoulders (scapulae) back together.
- Bring legs under the bar.
- Bring feet and hips into selected stance.
- Stand erect.
- Step back and clear racks.

Descent

- Take a deep breath and expand the chest.
- Tighten the latissimus dorsi.
- Release the gluteus.
- Draw hips back and down.
- Pull knees out.
- Keep heels flat on the floor.

Ascent

- Lift sternum up and tighten abdominal wall.
- Fire gluteus muscles and hamstrings.
- Calves contract (gastrocnemius) along with the soleus.
- Quadriceps take the strain.
- Gluteus medius, maximus and minimus continue to emit power.
- Lumbar region contracts and holds a pivot point.
- Spinae erector and lattimus dorsi hold the torso vertical.
- Abdominals, including the obliquus externus, remain under tension throughout the lift.
- Lower part of body continues to take the strain, transmitting power through to the gluteus back to the upper part of the body until the lifter is standing erect.

Developing Technique

Stability under load is demonstrated when a lifter is able to control the bar and prevent it, and their limbs, from being pulled out of line by the forces that come into play. When performing a squat the position of the feet, hands and the bar on the back, combined with the plane through which the hips travel, all have a direct impact on the forces of gravity and the pull on the lifter during different phases of the lift. The lifter must learn to create a posture with their body frame to balance and move the weight evenly over the feet. That said, the heels take a lot of the force and work hard to balance the lifter; these sit directly under the shoulder blades at the start and finish of the lift.

The hips move away from the centre of gravity during the lift by drawing back and down. As the weight and lifter descend, the knees become stabilizers but, as the lifter descends further, they are in a precarious position since they are in a transition phase. Therefore, they must prevent the force of the bar's weight from allowing the knees to travel too far forward over the toes.

The lifter must become aware of their lifting style and the ramifications of this. For instance, a top British female lifter has one leg slightly longer than the other, and in order to adopt an efficient squat stance she devised an unequal toe alignment, with one foot facing forward and the other with the toes pointing outwards. The heels were positioned directly under the shoulder blades in line with each other. She went on to gain a European squat record.

If a lifter prefers the bar to be higher on the back for the squat they should maintain a tight upright torso throughout the lift. If they prefer the bar lower down, they will need to sit further back on the descent and tilt the torso slightly forward. For this style they must have a very strong lower back.

Ankle flexibility will have an impact on either style as there must be sufficient dorsiflexion (upward movement in the ankle) during the lower part of the descent; otherwise the lifter will be unable to maintain good form. If there is insufficient ankle flexibility, this will affect the stress load on the knees and change the angle of the pelvic tilt, all of which will pull the lifter out of line, making it extremely difficult to fight against the forces of gravity. As a result, the lifter could be pulled off balance by the weight, fail the lift and, potentially, incur injury.

In order to squat well a lifter must develop an athlete-specific (customized to them) skill set, optimize their biomechanical levers and ensure muscle development, balance and flexibility. They should also build in sufficient rest and recovery periods and, when required, demonstrate high levels of mental toughness.

It is a general belief that good squatters have outstanding quadriceps and a huge back. While this is true, the most efficient way to squat is to utilize the rear of the body, making it take the lead and the majority of the work load.

The squat is conducted by three quarters of the posterior chain and a quarter of the anterior muscle chain, which together generate the moving force. The main combinations of the posterior chain employed in the squat are the erector spinae which act as key stabilizers. The hamstrings, which play a major role, therefore need to be immensely strong. The ability to create a good degree of hip tilt, with the gluteus maximus and adductor magnus acting as synergists, is paramount, as is first-rate ankle flexibility. The key anterior muscles are the quadriceps, which should be well formed, and the abdominals to act as antagonist stabilizers.

Powerlifting Squat Styles

There are two main styles of powerlifting back squat: medium-wide stance and narrow stance. The majority of lifters will naturally favour one over the other. Regardless of the chosen style for competition lifts, however, there is added value for the lifter to become proficient at all styles, as training the squat at different angles will improve the coordination of the different muscle groups. In turn this will aid both the lifter's body pro-perception and muscle adaptation. Thus, further growth and adaptation will be promoted by activating and varying muscular recruitment patterns simply by including different styles during a training cycle.

It is also important for the lifter to develop a sense of body awareness as this will enable them to feel when each muscle group has been activated during the course of the lift and help them identify when they are applying poor technique.

The squat styles share the same objective and follow the same movement, the aim being to take the bar from a standing position, break parallel and return to an upright position, although it should be noted that different muscle groups are recruited according to the style chosen.

Natural squatters are known to have a medium length torso and a slightly shorter leg span. These levers help the lifter to stay upright during the squat. The majority of lifters have to work hard over months and even years to produce a stance that helps them make the best of their biomechanical levers. To this end it is the medium-wide stance that is the most popular.

What is considered to be a medium stance by some lifters may be viewed as a wide stance by others. As a rule of thumb, if the feet are placed four to five inches wider than hip width apart, this would be relatively wide; some wide-stance lifters stand with their feet as wide apart as the bar sleeves. Whichever distance is preferred, for medium-wide stance the main emphases on muscle recruitment and the position of the bar on the back would be the same.

The ability to achieve a good wide stance depends on the degree of flexibility in the hip tilt and the strength and flexibility of the hip flexors, noting that foot placement is also dictated by this. The main attraction of the wide stance

is that the wider the stance, the less distance the bar has to travel.

Both medium and wide stances aim to keep the knees as close as possible to a right angle, which reduces some of the torque force on the knees. They also tend to have the bar positioned lower down the back. This makes it almost impossible not to have some degree of forward tilt, but the trade-off for the knees, gluteus recruitment and the reduced distance to travel is considered worthwhile. Moreover, if the lifter fails the squat or loses their grip with the bar positioned lower down the back, they are more likely to lose the bar behind them (as opposed to over the shoulders and head). This will increase the likelihood of the spotters catching the weight and so help to prevent injury.

Lifters with a shorter torso and/or longer legs naturally have a further distance to travel with the weight. Accordingly, they may opt for the narrow stance squat where the feet are placed with the outside of the foot in line with the middle to the outside of the shoulders. To descend in the narrow stance the knees are pushed forward and the hips kept vertical. This stance draws heavily on the quadriceps and lower lumbar region, as opposed to the hip flexors and hamstrings. Nevertheless, the load still needs to sit across the whole of the foot with the lifter using the heel of the foot as the base from which to push.

To help the lifter stay upright, as well as maintain balance and optimize the body's levers, the narrow stance requires the bar to be placed higher up the back, near the mid to upper trapezius muscles. While this higher placement throws a lot of force and strain onto the lower back, well-developed quadriceps can offset some of this weight distribution.

Grip
The hands should be positioned on the bar as close to each other as possible, without causing too much strain in the shoulders. The closer the grip, the easier it is to squeeze the

scapulae together and keep the erector muscles contracted, thereby creating a 'shelf' on which the bar can sit. However, this will be dictated by the flexibility of the shoulders and the pectoral muscles: flexibility is required in both areas. Some lifters have a grip as wide as the gap between the weights due to old shoulder injuries or upper back hypertrophy, while others have a grip as narrow as their own shoulder width.

Lifters can begin the set-up phase of the lift with their hands relatively wide, then as they warm up and move between their hands to take the bar from the racks they may readjust the hand spacing to bring them closer to the shoulders. They will need to maintain a strong grip and keep their fingers wrapped around the bar (where possible) for the duration of the lift.

Pelvis, hips and connecting hip flexors

The ability of the pelvis to tilt, and the degree to which this can be done, is paramount to human body posture. The degree of tilt and stability within the stance is directly linked to the hips. The hip joint sits next to the gluteal region, and rests below the iliac crest while overlying part of the femur (thigh bone), all of which are supported by the lower lumbar region. Thus, the hip is designed to support the body during standing, walking and running. In effect, it controls both movement and static posture.

Directly linked to the hips and pelvis are the hip flexors, a group of muscles which work in unison in order to mobilize the femur. When activated they control how the knee is pushed forward.

In powerlifting terms it is the pelvis that allows the hips to draw back and down to the full depth of the squat (below parallel). It is the hip flexors that stabilize the movement, define the width of the stance and influence how far the knee is pushed during the lift. As such, the performance of a successful squat relies on the ability to work the pelvic tilt and on having strong and flexible hip flexors.

Back

The back is attached directly to the abdominal wall. It is the kingpin of everything and performs two functions during the squat: firstly it supports the hips, the middle of the spine, the pelvic girdle and the trapezius, and secondly it must bear the weight that is sitting directly on it. As such, it must manage a huge amount of torque force (where the stress on the body is centred during a movement).

The upper back must be trained in relation to the weight it is expected to carry. Take, as an example, a woman with very soft, under-developed latissimus dorsi muscles who weighs 60kg and is holding 120kg on her back. She may well be strong enough to hold the weight, but without the appropriate muscle density, other parts of the body will have to take the strain, a role they have not been designed for. This can lead to serious injury.

The lower back (lumbar region) has a more complex role as it must fight against all the torque forces to avoid folding in the middle when squatting. This is an area that is sometimes neglected for leg work – some athletes spend more time training their legs than their lower back, but by training both, they could achieve a better stability under load.

If a lifter relies too much on a lifting belt during training, the lower back is unlikely to strengthen and adapt in line with the other muscles in the body since the belt will be doing too much of the work. As a result, when faced with a maximum load, the lower back becomes the weak link and can be overwhelmed by the force so that it folds and/or twists out of line, more often than not causing injury. The lifter may wonder why this is the case as they could have powerful legs capable of lifting up to 150 per cent more than what they were attempting to squat in competition. It is worth remembering here the traditional powerlifting saying: 'You are only as strong as your weakest link'.

A simple way to prevent weakness in the lower back is to delay using the belt by one to two sets later per training cycle. For instance, if the maximum weight the lifter can move is 100kg, they should use the belt when lifting 75kg. In the next training cycle they would use the belt at 80kg and so on, thereby progressively strengthening the back while ensuring it is properly supported when lifting the heavier weights. Alternatively, they could wear a looser belt on the first part of the warm-ups, encouraging the back to take some of the load while it is still being supported by the belt.

Legs

The squat is undoubtedly the most successful exercise for increasing muscle density in the legs. Deeper squats do activate muscles in the legs, yet good legs are required to squat in the first place so it is something of a chicken and egg situation. However it is viewed, the legs and the squat are intrinsically linked.

Opinions differ on the quadriceps-to-hamstring ratio required to perform the one-repetition maximum squat. Top powerlifting squatters tend to aim for a 35 per cent quadriceps to 65 per cent hamstring split as they need stronger hamstrings than quads, although it should be noted that the quadriceps of any powerlifter are going to be far more developed than the average person who trains with weights. Physiotherapists, on the other hand, would advocate a more equal split of power and development between and across the leg muscles.

The leg muscles span three main joints: hips, knees and ankles, their main function in the squat being to generate force and movement. The hamstrings are the prime mover (dynamic stabilizers) and promote explosive power and speed. They are essential for getting out of a deep knee bend squat. Good hamstrings also counteract the anteriority forces emitted from the quadriceps when performing the squat.

The quadriceps are generally recognized as the teardrop shaped muscle (vastus medialis) at the knees. As this is a four-headed muscle that covers the whole of the front of the thigh,

powerlifters do require first-rate quadriceps, including the inner and outer sweep of the leg (vastus medialis and vastus lateralis). The quadriceps generate huge power and form the shape of the stance of the squat, similar to the legs of a chair. They are imperative for the squat and largely support and hold the body in shape throughout. They can maintain a static position at the bottom of the squat whilst the gluteus and hamstrings contract, thereby enabling a powerful start to the ascent. At the same time they act as extensors for the knee joint. If the knees tend to come in during the squat this is likely to be due to weak quadriceps.

It should be remembered that powerlifting is a test of maximum strength. Good technique helps the lifter to lift more weight efficiently which, in turn goes a long way towards preventing injury. When a lifter has developed a sense of self and body awareness within the sport they will create and modify a lifting style that is unique to them. This will differ slightly according from where they are in their training programme and the equipment they are wearing. For example, they may squat slightly wider and more upright without a lifting suit.

All lifters can become proficient at the squat, and with consistent good technique they can build up a total through competition that enables them to achieve a respectable overall powerlifting total.

Preparing to Lift

1. Begin by standing at the centre of the loaded bar and an arm's length away. Place the hands on the bar and find your chosen grip. If the grip is too narrow to allow you to step within it, adjust accordingly.
2. Walk forward under the bar, keeping your hands in place. When your feet are parallel and directly under the bar, feel the bar with the trapezius muscles and nuzzle up to it. Bring the hands in if required and tighten the grip.

3. Fold the scapula together, brace the back and shoulders, maintain a tight grip, push up with the feet, pull the hips forward and stand upright with the bar. (Be sure to have the rack height low enough to clear the racks with the weight.) Look forward with eyes slightly upwards. Do not tilt the neck too far back or look down once the lift has begun. As you take the full weight you may feel compounded compression, as if the weight is actually pushing you down to the floor. This will settle.

4. When free standing with the loaded bar, lead with your heel and move your preferred leg back and out to the side so that you adopt a straddle position. When your foot is flat on the floor and the weight is stable, repeat the process with the other foot. The feet will now be in your chosen lifting stance.

5. Now that you are standing upright and clear of the squat racks, your knees must be seen to be locked out and the bar not too far down the back as you await the referee's signal to commence the lift. (See Federation rules for reasons not to be granted the start signal.) Once the referee is happy they will give the command 'Squat'.

6. Keep the eyes looking up (it may help to pick a spot on the wall and focus on this during the lift), take a big breath, bring the hips back and begin to draw the knees out while keeping the back tight and descend.

7. At this point you will naturally tilt forward so it is important to keep bracing the back against the bar to make a controlled descent. Resist folding in the middle and use the abdominal wall to push against the lifting belt. Tilt the hips down, not back, and continue to lead with them until they have dipped just below parallel with the knees. Do not let the weight push the knees too far over the foot.

8. Having broken parallel, tighten the gluteus maximus and push up and back. The knees will want to pull inwards but you should resist this and keep pushing them out. Now, lead with the chest, keep the head up and maintain the weight through the heels of the foot. Do not push through the toes as this will pull you forward. Keep pulling the bar into the back without letting it roll and you will begin to rise. Once out of the lower dip, bring the hips back in, draw the knees back and use all your leg strength to keep a solid platform and the weight moving upwards.

9. Keep pushing up and back and fight through the sticking point as any release of tension will cause the weight to drop. (The sticking point is where one muscle group takes over from another and can vary according to each lifter's muscle adaptation and skeletal alignment.)

10. Once standing fully erect wait for the referee to say 'Rack' and walk the bar back to the racks. Now walk forwards and dip slightly to place the bar back into the racks. Although the spotters can assist with replacing the weight you must not lose control of the bar until it is safely replaced in the squat racks.

11. Take extreme care to prevent your back twisting when taking and replacing the bar and ensure that the weight is balanced evenly throughout the movement. Always work with a training partner or someone who can spot for you. Whomever you choose, spend time getting to know them and allow them to understand you and become familiar with your weak areas. It would also be useful to identify if they have any previous injuries which may reduce their effectiveness as a spotter: you should know how much weight they can lift so that you are confident that they will be able to step in and help you avoid injury while preventing injury to themselves.

Sequence of Squat positions (front and side views)

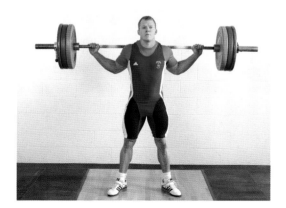

Squat Position A, front view.

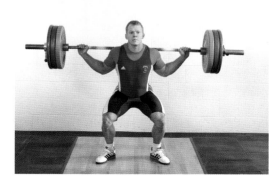

Squat Position B, front view.

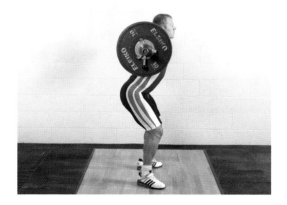

Squat Position B, side view.

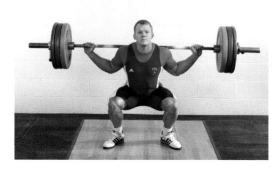

Squat Position C, front view.

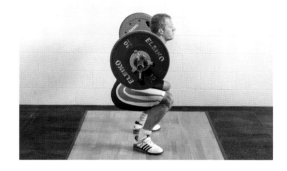

Squat Position C, side view.

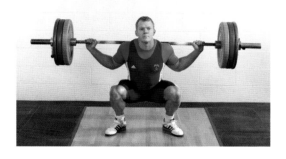

Squat Position D, front view.

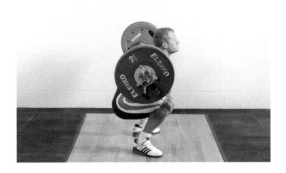

Squat Position D, side view.

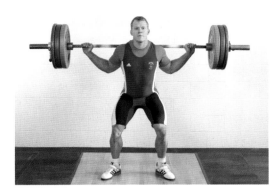

Squat Position E, front view (three quarters ascent).

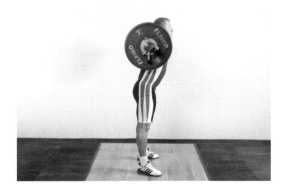

Squat Final Position, side view.

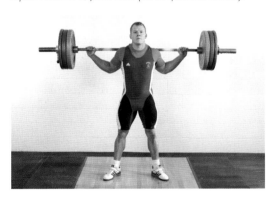

Squat Final Position, front view.

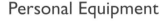

Personal Equipment

When competing in an equipped competition, lifters may choose to wear a combination of an erector shirt, super suit and wrist wraps, or they may opt to omit certain items if they feel they do not get enough performance outcome from them. However, if a lifter chooses to compete in an unequipped competition the only items permitted are a lifting belt and sometimes, but not always, knee wraps. A lifter may choose to lift in an equipped competition without the full lifting equipment, but they may not compete in an unequipped competition with a super suit or erector shirt.

It should be noted that all lifting attire, includ-ing support suits, shirts and wraps can only be worn in competition if the manufacturers have officially been registered and approved by the technical committee of the chosen powerlifting federation. These guidelines must be adhered to for all competitions from divisional level through to world championships. It should be noted that there may be differences between federations on the type, fabric, and make-up of lifting attire permitted.

Lifting singlet

In an unequipped powerlifting competition a one-piece lifting singlet must be worn. This should have no reinforced seams or panels and must be short in the legs (see the relevant federation rules for leg length and shoulder strap width). A short sleeved t-shirt should be worn under the singlet. This should be cotton and contain no more than 20 per cent elastane. Shorts and t-shirt (or any other double combinations) are not permitted, nor are long-legged suits of any type or tracksuit bottoms.

Squat suit

In equipped competitions special lifting suits known as super suits must be worn. These are cut from very strongly woven single-ply fabric that looks like canvas. Some suits are so rigid they actually stand up on their own. The seams in the suits, which are welded together or attached with iron clad thread, are strategically placed to simulate a harness around the anatomical levers of the hips and torso. Each manufacturer has a patented design according to where they believe is the most performance enhancing position for the seams to sit. The better quality suits have more stitching per square inch of fabric.

The lifter chooses their suit according to their body weight class, height and selected stance. If budget allows they can opt to have one custom made. Finding the right suit can be a matter of trial and error but a lifter will usually start with a softer, looser fitting suit and move on to a very tight type; top lifters' suits are so tight they can take up to forty minutes to put on, require assistance to do so and leave red marks when removed. Lifters often find that if a suit fits well around the hips and over the legs, they are too long in the torso and offer little support over the shoulders. To address this, the lifter may adapt the suit by inserting a seam across the top two inches on the shoulder straps, effectively making the suit shorter in the body.

If the suit fits well and the lifter has a technique to take full advantage of it, it acts as another set of erector muscles providing an intense feeling of added stability under load. A lifter can achieve an additional 50kg to 90kg on their squat by wearing a super suit, so it is worth spending the time and effort on choosing the correct type.

It can help to talk to other lifters who have a similar lifting style or body composition or who have plenty of experience with super suits. Irrespective of budget it is vital to go to a reputable supplier, as inferior suits have been known to 'blow out' or burst their seams at the bottom of the squat with the result that the suit ceases to offer the correct support. This can lead to serious injury.

Erector shirts

Erector shirts are, in effect, extremely tight closely woven t-shirts (they can be sleeveless) which are designed to give the impression of having an additional erector spinae muscle, hence the name. By pinning the shoulders back, they help the lifter stay upright during the squat thereby aiding stability and preventing them from folding partway through.

While erector shirts can enhance confidence and may be regarded as an extra safety measure for the lifter, there are mixed views on how effective they are in terms of preventing injury and increasing performance output. On the positive side, the shirt, when worn with a powerlifting suit, can make the lifter feel safely cocooned when they are lifting maximum weight on their back. However, the shirt can also make the lifter feel constricted within the upper trunk and chest cavity and unable to gain a deep full breath. The decision to wear a shirt comes down to a preference between feeling more able to fill up the chest cavity with air or accepting the constriction, perceived or otherwise, while gaining extra back support.

Wrist wraps

The wrist wrap holds the wrist in place when the lifter works to keep the bar in position on their back. Wrist wraps are identical to knee wraps in construction but are shorter: up to one metre in length and no wider than 8cm. They have an elastic loop at one end so that the lifter can attach this over the thumb and hold the wrap securely in place whilst binding the wrap around the wrist.

Belts

Lifters who wear a lifting belt appear to accelerate out of the bottom of the squat more quickly and efficiently than those who do not, and a belt is the first piece of equipment that a lifter will purchase. A belt produces increased pressure within the intra-abdominal wall so the lifter must learn to manage this pressure and lift with it. Having done so, the lifter will find that the belt helps to keep the spinal cord in alignment, enabling them to maintain a more erect position and reduce the likelihood of folding in on themselves during the squat. Since the lifter is more able to maintain correct form, the joint to muscle range of movement becomes less restricted and a more direct and efficient pathway is created for the bar to travel. In short, the lifter will reach the top of the squat more quickly by being manipulated into a good lifting position.

Knee wraps

Knee wraps are very important items of powerlifting equipment since they act as a reinforced set of tendons and protect the knee joint during the squat while enhancing the explosive power out of the bottom of the lift. They are usually purchased with a belt, and lifters can manage well for many years with these two items. Wraps are not obligatory in equipped competitions, but if used, they should be no longer than two metres in length and no wider than 8cm and should not be placed higher than the upper region of the thigh or low enough to cover the calf muscles. They can be wrapped in a spiral up and down the knee or in a criss-cross around the knee cap. Either style works well; the final choice is down to the individual lifter.

Top lifters often have three sets of knee wraps already rolled and held in place with an elastic band, one for each lift on platform. These can be hand-rolled (usually by the coach) or machine bound in a tight coil so that they can be wrapped as evenly and tightly as possible around the lifter's knee. The mechanical wrap machine can be helpful if a lifter does not have access to a coach

or training partner, although it requires some practice to apply the wraps without help. It is worth noting that if machine-wrapped wraps become uncoiled they can completely unravel and it can be time-consuming to rewrap them. Also, if a lifter has to use one hand-wrapped wrap and one that had been machine-wrapped this may cause a noticeable difference in the tension between the two knees which could adversely affect the line of the squat.

Leggings

As lifting suits are so tight, it can be very time-consuming to put one on. This can eat into valuable training time or competition warm-up time. Moreover, if a lifter puts the suit on with the seams in the wrong place or askew, they will not be able to get the full benefit. Specialized leggings help lifters save time and energy when putting on their suits. Made from a fine silky-feel fabric, they are supplied as single 'legs', each with a stirrup to hold the legging in place. The lifter pulls the legging on and the lifting suit goes on over the top. Once the suit is on high over the hips the leggings can be pulled off.

Socks

Socks must be worn and should not include logos that have not been approved by the chosen lifting federation. If long, they should not come into contact with the knee wraps.

Shoes and boots

Shoes or boots aid stability and reduce the chance of injury as the lifter pushes through their feet. The choice is down to the individual lifter who will be influenced by the degree of flexibility they have in their ankles and the level of comfort required. Shoes and boots are generally made of leather and have incompressible, non-slip soles which ensure that the lifter's body weight, together with the load on their back, is distributed evenly across the whole foot. The upper part of the shoe is firm yet pliable and is reinforced with one to two straps strategically placed across the top of the foot. The shoes have a built-in arch support which can aid the line of the hips and knees as they move in and out of the squat movement.

Lifters who favour the bar lower on their back fare better with a flatter shoe due to the altered pull of gravity. This type of shoe can be made of heavy canvas. With a flatter shoe lifters advocate they feel more in contact with the floor and in tune with their natural stance, making them feel more in control.

Chalk and resin

Chalk is used to stop the hands slipping on the bar during warm-ups and on the competition lifting platform. It comes in different compositions. Traditional weightlifting chalk can be a little too smooth for powerlifters, many of whom prefer to use climbing chalk. However, others prefer to use a resin which is moist when applied but which dries extremely quickly. Again the lifter will decide which they prefer. As powerlifters' hands become accustomed to the bar and develop calluses around the grip they predomi-

nantly train with, chalk becomes a tool for use in competition and when performing top lifts. Many gyms today prefer lifters to use resin as opposed to chalk as it is less messy. Both chalk and resin are easily available.

Smelling salts

Many powerlifters use smelling salts or ammonia capsules during competition or a heavy training session, believing this helps them take more oxygen into the lungs and thereby develop a larger, tighter torso and an improved body shape under load. However, this could be a placebo effect or a diversionary tactic: the sensory shock of the salts' strong smell may simply divert the lifter's thoughts away from the heavy weight they are about to lift. The warmer the smelling salts become, the more potent they become, so as the tonnage increases during a session, the stronger the salts will seem. While there may be little scientific basis to validate the use of such sensory aids, they are undeniably popular within the powerlifting community.

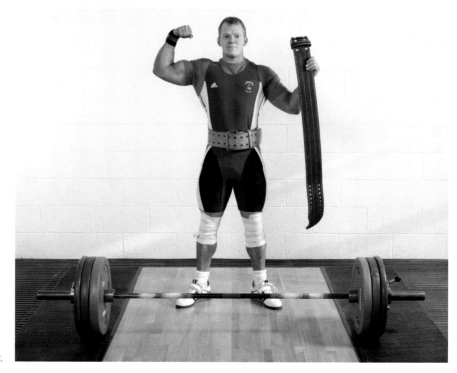

*Athlete wearing
personal equipment.*

CHAPTER 2

THE BENCH PRESS

The bench press is regarded as the greatest test of upper body strength and is highly popular with bodybuilders and strength athletes throughout the world. In powerlifting competitions it is performed after the squat and before the deadlift, and it is the lift most often executed at single lift competitions. It has been a Paralympic sport since 1984 (see later in this chapter).

As with the squat and the deadlift, the bench press is a closed skill sport, meaning that the lifter performs the same movement every time in a largely stable environment while controlling the amount of weight they want to lift. As with the other two lifts, the essence of the bench press lies in power, skill and technique. There is a distinct difference in this context between skill (a lifter's ability to understand and react to their environment) and technique (the systematic procedure they follow to execute the lifting task).

To excel in powerlifting an athlete who is

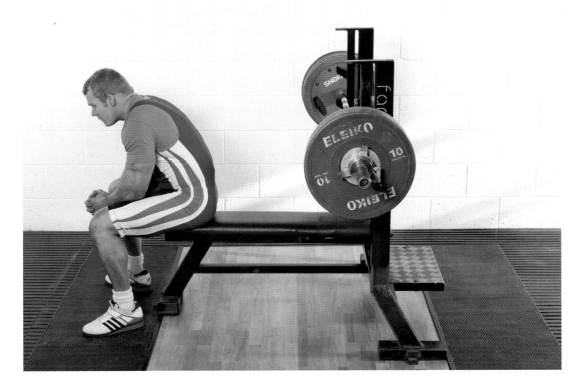

At rest.

strong in the squat and the deadlift must also become skilled in the bench press. However, it is often the case that the bench press receives less attention in training than the other two lifts. This is because, with the focus of the bench press being predominantly on the upper body, using the legs as stabilizing agents, the weight being pressed is less than in the squat and deadlift, which predominantly use the legs and back. So, while the total weight lifted in the bench press contributes to the overall total of the three lifts, it does not help to improve the individual totals of the squat or deadlift. However, if an athlete increases the weight they lift on the squat, they also increase what they can lift on the deadlift, and vice versa. As a result, the total weight lifted may increase significantly. For this reason some athletes regard the bench press as separate discipline from the other two lifts.

Performing the Bench Press

The bench press is executed lying on a gym bench with the lifter's head, shoulders and hips aligned on the bench and the feet flat on the floor. Once in position, the lifter takes hold of a loaded bar with elbows locked and, keeping the bar under control, bends the elbows and lowers it slowly to the chest. After pausing with the bar held motionless on the chest, the lifter pushes or 'presses' the bar back to its original starting point until the arms are straight and the elbows are locked once again. There are many views on how to achieve a successful bench press but here we propose that the real secret lies in positioning the body correctly on the bench before pressing heavy weights. (An explanation of how this can be best achieved appears later in the chapter.)

Anatomy

As with the squat and the deadlift, a lifter is physically vulnerable when performing the bench

press and risks serious injury or even death if they do not train properly. Therefore, as with the other two lifts, it is important to have a basic understanding of anatomy (how the body is structured) and biomechanics (how bones, muscles, tendons and ligaments work together to produce movement). This will help the lifter and their coach decide how the body should be positioned and how it must be made to move in order to ensure the most appropriate training programme is developed. The ultimate goal is to ensure that the bench press is executed safely and to maximum effect.

Spine

The skeletal shape influences the lifter's posture on the bench and the alignment of their spine along the centre of the bench. If a lifter has scoliosis (curvature of the spine), their position on the bench will be off kilter, so they will need to modify their grip on the bar and the placement of their shoulders and hips to compensate for this.

Chest

The sternum and the pectoral girdle also play central roles in the bench press. There is a direct relationship between the position of the sternum and the point at which the bar sits once it has been lowered to the chest. If the lifter chooses to arch their back (see Developing Technique later in this chapter), the sternum should be raised and held in that position throughout the lift. It should be noted that the anatomical function of the sternum is to protect vital organs such as the heart and lungs. This serves as a reminder of how hazardous a bench press can be if strict form is not adhered to. Meanwhile the pectoral girdle serves as a major attachment point for all the relevant muscles that are linked to the shoulders and elbows, which in turn allows the engineering of movement during the lift to happen.

Elbows

The position of the elbows is very important in the bench press. Unless a bench shirt is being worn or narrow grip exercise is being performed, the optimal movement is to pull the elbows wide and directly apart from one another. This must be conducted with the elbows in parallel to one another. As the elbows pull apart and the bar begins to descend towards the chest it is important for the lifter to maintain a continuous tempo instead of allowing the bar to freefall towards the chest at any point in the descent. It is all about momentum – if a bar comes down too fast, it is like an out-of-control train and will crash. The lifter's aim is to achieve a smooth transition at every stage of the lift.

After taking the weight of the bar with locked (straight) arms, the lifter bends their elbows to start the downward phase of the lift. At this point they may experience a lot of sway which could cause them to hesitate, forcing them to hold the bar for longer and potentially causing loss of concentration. Nevertheless, the lifter must gain control of the bar and maintain a stable lifting position. A good analogy for this feeling is to imagine that the palms of the lifter's hands are similar to a novice ice skater's feet when first learning to skate on ice: both individuals struggle to find balance and maintain grip at the same time. As the lifter strives to achieve this their hands may want to slip apart due to the forces of gravity or perspiration, even when chalk has been used on the hands. To offset this feeling the lifter must continue to push the sternum up and lead the elbows out and away from the body, allowing the bar to descend to the chest and maintaining the skeletal shape they created as the structural basis of the lift.

To promote the upward phase of the bench press the elbows must begin to straighten and move back in towards the body. It is important to maintain control here as the heavy weights can pull the elbows out of line and place the lifter at risk of injury. At the same time, the wrists must remain straight (not bent backwards or forwards) and in direct line with the forearm throughout.

Shoulders

The scapulae (shoulder blades) sit on the rear side of the rib cage and act as a pivot which releases the sternum, enabling it to protrude upwards and allowing the shoulders to move without impingement. When a bench press is being performed the shoulder blades create a vital platform of stability for the torso. In turn this enables the arms to become the fulcrum that sits across an axis, meanwhile allowing the levers to become mobile within the framework of instability created by the continuous changing centre of gravity as the bar travels during the press movement. By creating dynamic control of movement the body becomes a tool with which to counterbalance the length and weight of the powerlifting bar.

A major component in all this is the group of four muscles

Demonstration of elbows in line with scapulae.

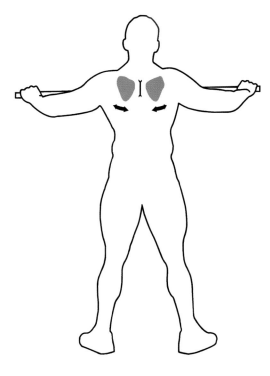

Vertical scapulae indentation line (showing scapulae drawing together).

This can force the shoulders to move too far forward, so that they come out of the frame of the shoulder girdle when the lifter pushes the bar back up from the chest, and this in turn can cause the bar to twist, leading to torn shoulder ligaments.

As with the squat and the deadlift, the aim in the bench press is to achieve efficient, smooth, compact and, above all, safe movements. Therefore a basic understanding of how the body works to achieve this is important.

known as the rotator cuff. This controls rotation of the shoulder and maintains stability in the joint by preventing the humerus (upper arm bone) from sliding out of its cavity. Bench press specialists are vulnerable to rotator cuff injury which can be caused by benching maximum load with too wide a grip. However, since this has the benefit of reducing the distance that the bar has to travel, some lifters feel it is worth the trade-off.

Another area of vulnerability for bench press specialists is a muscle imbalance caused by over-development of the pectoral muscles, both major and minor, and under-development of the rhomboid (located between the shoulder blade and the spine) and of the infraspinatus (one of the rotator cuff muscles, located behind the shoulder and covering the shoulder blade).

THE BENCH PRESS MOVEMENT

Creating a stable starting position

- Select the preferred grip.
- Lie prone on the bench.
- Adopt back shape (arch or flat).
- Place feet on the floor.
- Lock elbows and draw shoulders back into the bench.
- Take bar at arm's length.

Bar descent

- Tighten shoulders (rear deltoids and scapulae).
- Tighten gluteals.
- Lift up sternum.
- Maintain contraction on lower lumbar region.
- Bring bar down to chest.
- Keep feet on the floor.

Bar ascent

- Tighten the gluteals and the hamstrings.
- Push the feet into the floor.
- Push through the back (latissimus dorsi) and biceps.
- Keep lower lumbar region contracted.
- Release the shoulders (without lifting off the bench).
- Move the elbow joints.
- Push up through the triceps and forearms to lockout position.

Developing Technique

The essential technique components of a competition bench press are the grip (positioning of the hands on the bar), the back, the arch and the ability to maintain stability under load.

Bench press grip

The term 'grip' refers to the distance between the hands on a powerlifting bar. A lifter must select their grip before attempting to press weights and should maintain the grip throughout the lift. If the lifter is not competing, the grip will vary according to the muscle group being trained at any one time. For example, a narrow grip bench press is devised to place more emphasis on the triceps while reducing the effort from the chest, meaning that the distance between the hands is shorter. A medium grip, where the hands are further apart, will train the chest while, at the other end of the spectrum, a wide grip bench press, where the hands are further apart, is an exercise that works the outer range of muscles and thus tilts the intensity of the movement onto the shoulders. While the selection of grip will depend very much on the muscle group being exercised and, to a lesser extent, on the lifter's anatomy, it is important to note that, in competition, the International Powerlifting Federation rules state that the hands cannot be spaced more than 81cm apart, with the measurement taken from the index finger.

Competition bars have grip marks to help lifters place their hands in the correct position. Regardless of the chosen grip, the palms, fingers and thumbs should be fully wrapped around the bar before a lift is attempted (unless the relevant lifting federation states that a thumbless grip is permitted). It should be noted that the International Powerlifting Federation and International Paralympics Committee prohibit a thumbless grip in competition, and it is not recommended as part of a training programme since it reduces control of the bar and is potentially hazardous.

The lifter should take time to find the correct grip, primarily to prevent injury but also to enable more weight to be lifted. As a rule, individuals in similar weight classes have similar grips since they are likely to have similar bone structure, although bone density may vary. A lifter's anatomical grip is measured by taking a view of their skeletal frame. Of course, every skeleton is unique and there are small differences between male and female. However, when it comes to selecting a grip, the choices made by either sex are likely to be determined by the width, breadth, density of the fingers and shoulder girdle rather than physical strength or grip marks on the lifting bar. The gender gap is bridged with the female grip being a finger and a half closer than the male counterpart. To measure similarities for male and female, a rule of thumb is that a female of a similar height and frame to a male is likely to be up to three weight classes lighter than that of her male counterpart. So, a female weighing in at the 67.5kg class and a man weighing in at the 90kg class could both have similar grip spacing on the bar.

A biomechanical view should also be taken into account when choosing the grip. This involves assessment of muscle density and attachments and the development of the associated tendons. The density and arrangement differ according to the years of training, types of injury incurred and the amount and placement of subsequent scar tissue incurred in various muscles. This will all have an impact on the selection of grip. It should be noted that muscle growth can alter the biomechanical grip over time.

The biomechanical and anatomical views, when considered separately and together, give a good indication of a lifter's optimum grip. More often than not this is one and a half times longer than the width of the shoulder, noting that the actual measurement comes from the length of the clavicle (collarbone) and the girth of the muscle attached.

Until the lifter becomes proficient in selecting the appropriate grip it would be useful to enlist the help of a spotter who will guide the hands into the desired position on the bar before they pass the bar to them. An uneven grip can lead

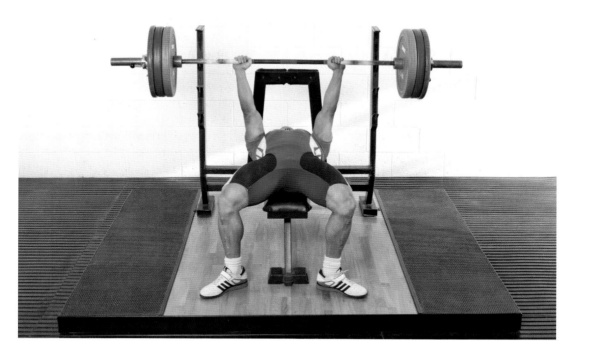

Narrow grip bench start position.

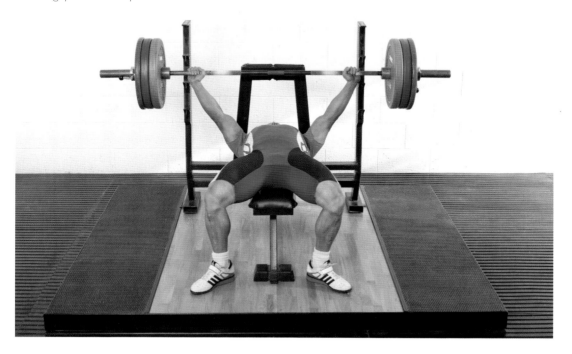

Wide grip bench start position.

to the lifter being unable to control the weight successfully.

Back

The back is the foundation of the bench press discipline by the very nature of its muscle mass compared to that of the chest, although many lifters place their focus on the chest, believing that this is what really drives the lift. As such, the back is frequently overlooked in training or not trained as intensely as warranted. There is a saying within the world of weights, 'Big bench means big chest', but this can be misconstrued – does a lifter need a big chest to achieve a credible powerlifting press or does the bench press movement itself create an impressive set of pectoral muscles? The chicken and egg scenario comes to mind here. In the powerlifting arena the majority of top lifters would probably agree that it is all about the back, chest, shoulders and triceps, in that order. The back acts as the stabilizing agent that makes it possible for the chest muscles to press the weight. Imagine a 'sandwich', with the back muscles acting as the base layer, the spine sitting in the middle and the chest muscles providing the top layer. While beginners and intermediate lifters will work to establish a good all-round muscle base and a solid technique, a top bench presser would refocus their training onto major back workouts.

More advanced lifters assess their control and power output to enable them to identify their weak links and design their training sessions to address these in a way that suits their own bench press style, for example the order in which they train specific groups of muscles such as those of the back, for example the infraspinatus, the teres major, the teres minor, rhomboid and the latissimus dorsi. This does not mean the chest becomes dormant, however. It is similar to having a good set of stabilizers on a bike: they play an important role and need maintaining but it is the main wheels that are the driving force and warrant most attention. The focus on the back in the bench press is mainly due to the fact that it is the largest single muscle group involved.

In order to cover the same area and mass to trigger the same power output, the chest must enlist the help of the abdominals. This is not an issue on its own but it can be isolated when assessing the economy of muscle to power ratio (the amount of force that the muscle can produce). On the basis of size, volume and relative force generated, therefore, the back wins.

While it is, of course important to strengthen all the muscle groups during training, the lifter must also develop the ability to 'pull' and 'push' in order to achieve a controlled bench press. To explain, pulling is the act of bringing the weight down under control towards the chest, while pushing or 'pressing', as the term suggests, is the act of pushing the weight up and away from the body. The term 'puller' is usually associated with the deadlift, while 'pusher' is derived from bench pressing.

Arch

Top bench press specialists often strive to create a massive arch in their back when they bench press as this can shorten the distance the bar has to travel towards and away from the chest. This should not be taken as a given, however, since the arch does not suit all lifters and caution should be exercised, particularly if the lifter has a history of back pain or an injury.

The major factor in developing a pliable yet stable arch is the ability to work with the spinae (skeletal spine). Also important are the abdominals. The rectus abdominis (upper abdominals) warrant particular attention, mainly due to their direct placement near the sternum. The obliquus externums, (abdominal muscles on the torso) are also important as they help to 'bind' everything together and also aid stabilization. There may be some focus on these areas in the lifter's training programme, but quite often it is insufficient attention to make the abdominals a prominent component of the arch or the body shape that the lifter works so hard to formulate for the big bench press. It takes time and dedication to create the muscle, relative attachments

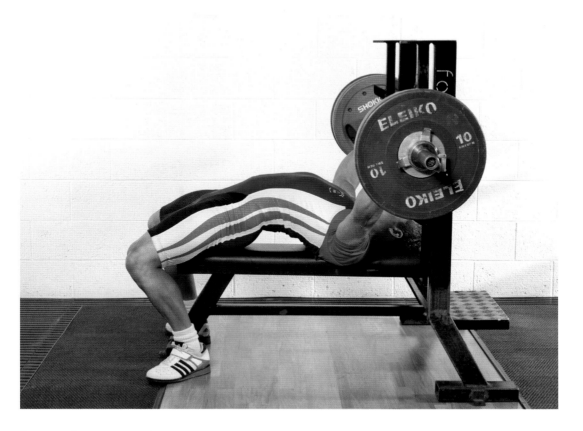

Side view of bench press arch.

and insertions to build and sustain an arch position for the bench press. Once achieved, though, the arch can be maintained for years and is the tool of many a world champion.

Stability under load

Stability under load is now a major factor, as if the bar cannot be controlled there is a high chance that it will pull the lifter to one side or another. In extreme circumstances, the lifter may lose control to the point of letting the bar drop and risking serious injury as a result. Bench press competition rules state that before the start signal can be granted for a lift, the bar should be held and locked out at arm's length. If the lifter cannot stabilize the bar in the way

required before beginning the descent phase of the lift, the adjudicating referee is unable to give the start signal. There is a time restriction involved here as the lifter only has sixty seconds to commence the lift. If stability cannot be demonstrated within this time limit the referees are obliged to show three red lights and the result is an unsuccessful attempt.

If the signal is granted, but for whatever reason stability under load starts to reduce, it becomes harder for the lifter to keep the bar following the correct pathway. Some lifters have an excellent lock-out position and may gain the start signal only to lose control of the bar as it nears the halfway point of the descent, a situation that may only come into play as the weight on the bar increases. Often the lifter thinks the loss of stability is down to lack of strength but, in reality, it is more likely to be linked to the number and combination of weights used to load the bar as the tonnage increases. Consider the scenario where a lifter who is excellent at lifting 135kg falters when attempting 140kg, even though they can perform numerous repetitions at 135 kg during training. More often than not this is due to the lifter's coach omitting to take into account the progressive loading of the bar in competition and the knock-on effects this has. For example, to increase the load on the bar from 135 kg to 140 kg, some of the smaller discs already in place would be removed from the bar and a pair of large 25kg discs added to create the total of 140kg, instead of simply using two 2.5kg discs to provide the extra 5kg. This new combination of discs could be enough to affect both the centre of gravity and how the lifter moves the bar at the different stages of its pathway.

As discussed in the squat chapter, stability under load needs to be counterbalanced. In this instance an easy remedy would be to train with discs similar to those used in competition. This would take into account the actual composition of the discs: the majority of powerlifting competitions use cast iron weights, making them narrower than those typically used in training, which are often coated with rubber and vary according to the manufacturer's design. Sometimes rubber-coated discs are used in competition, and on large tonnage this can increase the space they take up on the bar, altering the forces of pull against the lifter. If this differs from what the lifter has become used to in training, it can result in too much sway in the bar for the lifter to fight against, culminating in a failed lift.

It is also worth noting that, while many gyms use spring-loaded collars to hold the discs in place, as a safety precaution full collars are used in competitions for this purpose. These are longer and wider than their spring-loaded counterparts and weigh 2.5kg each, thereby altering the combination of weights on the bar and potentially changing the forces of gravity that come into play. Since they are required to be used in competition, they should be used in training.

Even taking all these factors into account, further work may be required to create a stable platform from which to bench. As mentioned earlier, this is mainly due to the fact that in a bench press scenario, the body is in effect a mechanical system that is aligned to create a fulcrum, not only to create balance but also to work against the force of the huge weights being pressed. Success in the bench press depends on the ability to keep the body shape in line with the directional forces that define the pathway of the bar. The key is to go with gravity and not fight it any more than absolutely necessary. To do this well the lifter needs good proprioception (awareness of the position of the body) and the ability to understand and control individual muscle groups. They also require a cognitive understanding of the role that the tendons play. This understanding will allow the lifter to control their arm movement within the optimal parameters of their own anatomy so that strength and force can be called into play to bring the bar back into line when needed. Imagine a top-heavy tree that looks strong and stable on a fine, sunny day but topples over in a big storm. The same goes for the powerlifter who, under comfortable weights but with some instability, will be able to lift the weight out of line. But once under heavy tonnage, for example at 90 per cent and above of the lifter's One Rep Max (the maximum weight they can achieve, often referred to as 1RM), the weakness begins to show to the point that the bar is forced either too far forward near the abdominals and the lifter loses control or the bar falls towards the neck and, again, control is lost and consequently so is the lift.

Passing the bar

There are two ways in which the bar can be passed to the lifter: a side pass or a centre pass. A side pass is where two loaders stand at oppo-

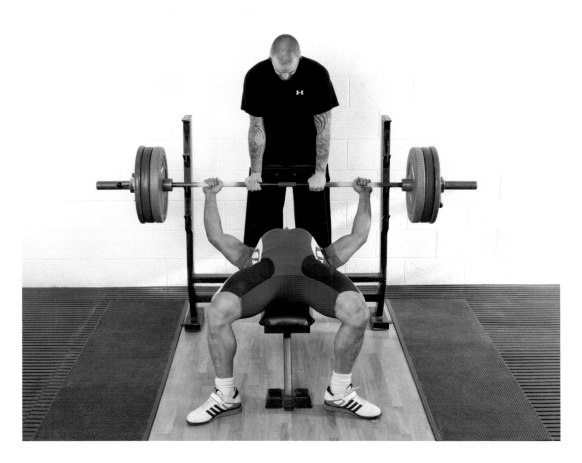

Passing the bar for the bench press.

site ends of the bar and pass the bar directly to the lifter's hands. A centre pass is where one loader stands behind the lifter's head and passes the bar to them. The way in which the bar is passed to the lifter has a direct effect on how they cope with instability when first taking the load. For example, if the bar is passed from the centre and the loader is not strong enough to pass it evenly to the lifter, this will affect the handover and the lifter will have to adjust to the imbalance. Similarly, if one of the loaders on a side pass releases the bar too quickly, it will result in an imbalance and, again, the lifter must quickly adjust. Both types of pass

can be uneven and one is no better or worse than the other. The best option is to train using both methods.

Within the context of stability under load, the term 'pulling' refers to realigning the bar into the correct position at arm's length following the handover. A typical scenario would be when the bar is handed to the lifter too early, resulting in it sitting closer to the neck and shoulders than at the highest point of the chest, where it should be. The lifter must then take the full weight and pull it into the correct line before attempting to bring the bar down to the chest.

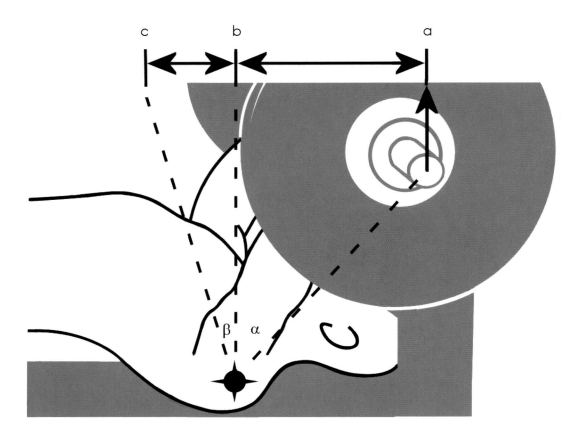

Bench press depicting angles of safety.

Preparing to Lift

Having considered all the elements that contribute to a successful bench press, it is now time to join all the dots and explain how to set up a bench press position.

1. Start by straddling the bench, positioning yourself approximately three quarters of the way down the bench.
2. Imagine that you are about to squat and lower yourself onto the bench, leading with the hips and tilting them slightly backwards.
3. Sit down on the bench with the feet parallel to each other and flat on the floor, toes slightly pointing outward.

4. If you feel for any reason that a full extended arch position created by concaving the spine is either not suitable due to flexibility issues (possible previous injuries) or is not advantageous due to the design of the chosen bench shirt, adopt a more prone approach (known as a flat back position). Here, only the sternum is slightly raised as opposed to the whole lumbar region, as would be seen in an arched position. To execute this, gently but firmly place the spine down the middle of the bench. Lift the sternum slightly and push the rest of the spine and hips into the bench, keeping the feet flat on the floor, creating a firm base. Now stretch your arms to full length above your head and place

your hands in the correct grip position on the bar.

Whichever position you have chosen, proceed following steps 5 to 8.

5. If you have chosen an arched position 'walk' the shoulders down the bench towards the lower spine, then lift them off the surface of the bench. As a lever to help with this you can use the powerlifting bar (which should always be loaded on the racks before you start) or the struts of the bench at the side. Alternatively, if you have a shorter reach, use the bench itself. Whichever option you choose, push against it with the hands and push up through the feet and hips.
6. Relax the trapezius (shoulder and upper back) muscles in order to bring the scapulae back towards each other. Imagine you are trying to make the gap between the shoulder blades smaller.
7. Draw the feet further back towards the gluteus maximus (buttocks), going onto the balls of the feet for more leverage.
8. Once the arch has been established place the feet flat on the floor, realign the shoulders and head back on the bench and place the hands in the correct grip position, taking care to ensure that the arch shape is maintained. (Note that, in a competition scenario, the top of the head must not extend beyond the end of the bench.)

Once everything is locked into place, with the feet flat on the floor, the head, scapulae and buttocks in contact with the bench and a good solid grip established, you will have constructed 'the elected body position' and will be ready to take the weight at arm's length and begin the lift.

Sequence of competition bench press movements.

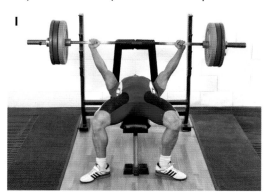

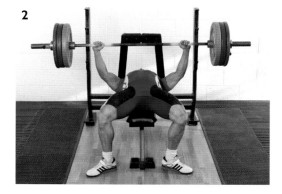

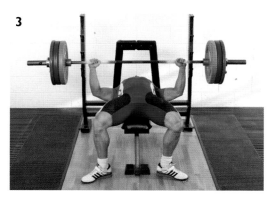

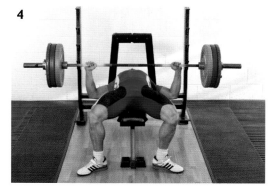

5

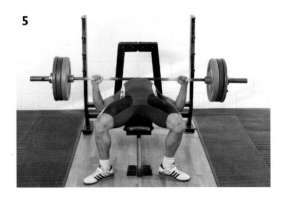

6

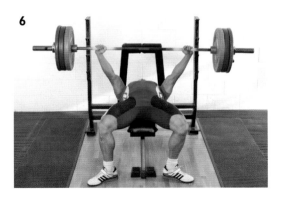

Sequence for narrow grip bench press.

1

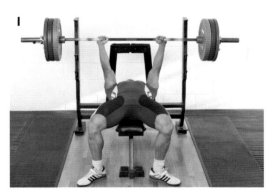

2

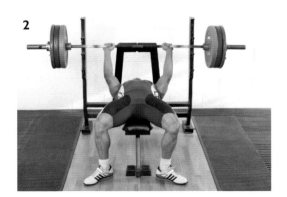

3

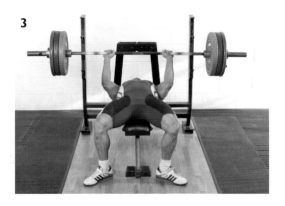

4

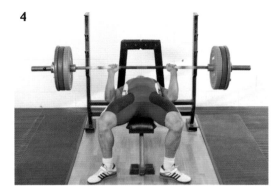

5

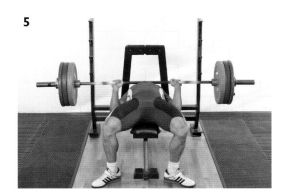

6

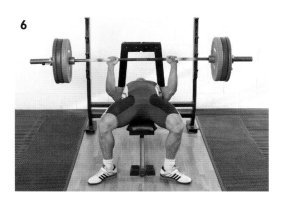

7

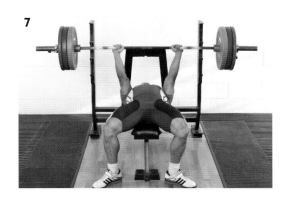

Sequence for wide grip bench press.

1

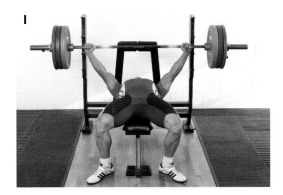

2

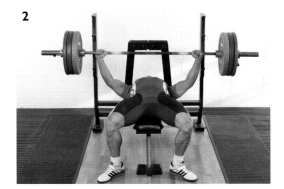

3

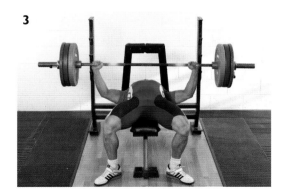

4

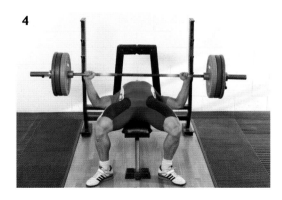

5

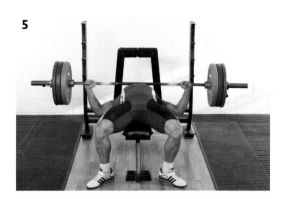

6

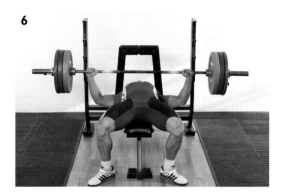

7

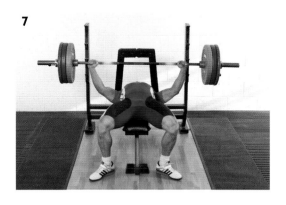

8

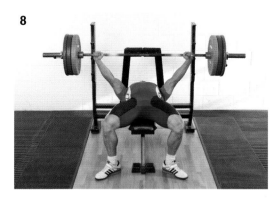

Paralympics Bench Press

Powerlifting for athletes with a disability consists solely of the bench press. This discipline stands as a sport in its own right, and its athletes achieve world and Paralympic records equal to, and often exceeding, non-disabled equivalent bench press records. The rules for IPC bench press align as closely as possible to the mother sport of IPF powerlifting which comprises the three lifts: squat, bench press and deadlift.

The 'bench press specialist' discipline is considered to be the ultimate test of upper body strength and mental toughness. It sits within British weightlifting and links into the British Paralympic Association (BPA) in the same way that weightlifting links into the British Olympic Association (BOA). Above this, the sport is placed within the International Paralympic Association (IPC) which currently takes the role of the international federation for the sport of Paralympic powerlifting and is the key reference point for rules, international ranking lists, all regulations for international events and eligibility for competing at the Paralympic Games. Each Paralympic cycle runs for four years, in the same way as the Olympics, while each World Championships and European cycle runs for two years.

There are up to 200 countries participating within this area, all with lifters at various attainment levels, from recreational participants to world class performers. Top lifters are currently lifting more than three and a half times their own body weight. In the London 2012 Games a Nigerian male lifter weighing in at the under 48kg class successfully lifted 180kg.

GB at the Paralympic Games

Great Britain has an excellent history of success for the bench press within the Paralympics. Women powerlifting bench pressers were first permitted to compete at the Sydney Games in

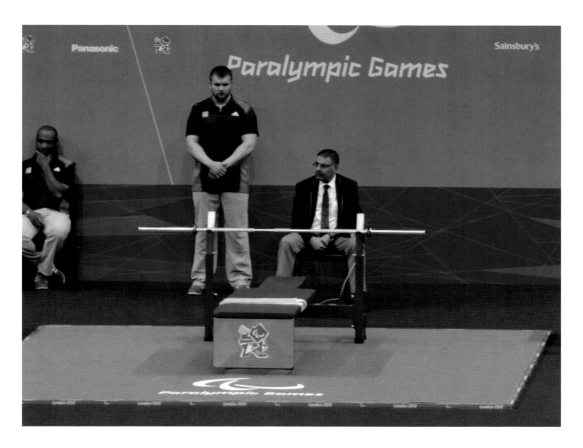

The Paralympic bench press at the London 2012 Paralympic Games.

2000. It was here that the British athlete, Emma Brown, won a gold medal and set a Paralympics record (adding to her collection of world records). She followed this up by gaining her second Paralympics gold medal in the Athens Games in 2004. Emma was unbeaten in international competition for thirteen consecutive years.

Alongside Emma at the Sydney Games, Anthony Peddle, another British lifter, won a gold medal and set a record that was to stand for many years, lifting 168kg in the under 48kg class. Anthony went on to lift in seven Paralympic Games - no easy feat as you must be ranked within the top ten in the world to be selected. Jason Irving was to take up the mantel for Team GB, gaining a silver medal in the Commonwealth Games in 2006, and just losing out on a medal in Beijing 2008.

In the London 2012 Games, Briton Zoe Newson won a bronze medal at the young age of twenty, while Ali Jowad just lost out on a silver medal. Powerlifting is a growing sport in Great Britain in terms of popularity and level of achievement. It is worth noting that the totals required to gain medals at a Paralympic Games is ever-increasing. Great Britain currently has very talented athletes entering the world class programme, all of whom have excellent potential to become world class athletes.

For IPC powerlifters to gain funding they must achieve the set qualifying standard. This is ultimately set by the British Paralympic Association in conjunction with UK Sport. The required lifting total is formulated on the predictability of the individual winning a medal at a Paralympic Games. Funding increases the closer to medal potential and medal colour (bronze, silver, or gold) the lifter is deemed to be. Therefore, a gold medallist at the previous Games, who is fit and fully committed to train, is likely to be awarded the highest tier of funding that the sport has to offer. Likewise, if they obtain the minimum standard which indicates potential for the sport at elite level the funding award would be the minimum. Hence, funding has a direct link to performance output. As an athlete progresses, the funding they could receive increases accordingly.

This funding and entry on to a world class programme facilitates arrangements for the athlete's event calendar and sporting pathway to success in that it subsidizes travel, accommodation and competition entry fees. Primarily, funding allows athletes to spend more time training, recovering and competing while granting access to top coaches, service providers and technological research and development.

At a Paralympic Games there can only be one athlete representing their country in each weight class, as opposed to two in world championships and below. IPF currently is not an Olympic sport; therefore a world championships is the highest ranked event.

Once selected for a Paralympic Games the powerlifter becomes part of a larger organization: Team GB. Consequently they are subject to all the rules and regulations of the British Paralympic Association and the LOC (Local Organizing Committee of the Olympic and Paralympic Games). Accordingly, the athletes must sign a comprehensive contract for Team GB, as well as a sport-specific contract. Each contract includes very clear instructions relating to sponsorship and product endorsement, codes of behaviour, both on and off field of play. They will be made acutely aware of all responsibilities linked to receiving funding.

At the same time, the athlete becomes part of a huge, life-defining and life-changing event. It is an event that many aspire to. Yet, in reality, relatively few athletes are actually selected to go to the Paralympics and even fewer go on to become medallists. Accordingly, the powerlifter is granted the same opportunities to succeed as any athlete from the other Paralympic and Olympic sports. They are invited to holding and preparation camps where all the top athletes across all the sports train together to prepare for the Games. They are able to attend seminars and talks, receive input from top service providers and share in the experiences of medal winners.

Paralympic powerlifters are in a unique position since their non-disabled IPF power-lifting counterparts do not have the opportunity compete at the Olympic Games. On entry to the Paralympics powerlifters are issued with full Team GB kit (which is additional to and different from their sport-specific kit). They are invited to attend the opening and closing ceremonies. They reside in the Paralympic village and are attract high levels of media attention. For this reason they are given intense training in living in a high pressure multi-sport environment where they will be sharing the same food hall and recreational facilities as the world's most famous athletes and coping with village life away from family and friends.

As Paralympians, the athletes reach the pinnacle of their sport; they come to understand the true meaning of excellence and to personify the Paralympic motto of 'Spirit in motion' and values of pride, inspiration and determination.

Differences between IPF powerlifting and IPC rules and equipment

Where possible the same rules are applied to both IPF and IPC powerlifting. The differences that occur are disability-specific. For example, all IPC athletes compete with their feet and lower body on an adapted bench, whereas in IPF the athletes are expected to place their feet on the floor or on blocks.

IPC powerlifting is part of the Paralympic movement and Team GB. Accordingly, IPC powerlifting is also part of the Olympic movement. As such it comes under Team GB and is therefore subject to all of the same rules, behaviours, expectations and contracts as every Olympic and Paralympic team that represents Great Britain in an Olympic and Paralympic Games. IPF powerlifting, as a non-Olympic sport, is currently only answerable to the rules of the International Powerlifting Federation and any contractual agreements they have reached

with their sponsors or organizing committees to ratify world ranking events.

All IPC powerlifters are required to have an IPC licence and an appropriate classification status (see classification below). This system is does not apply to IPF.

Within the rules of play once their name has been called by the competition announcer an IPC athlete is granted two minutes to commence their lift, instead of one minute for an IPF athlete.

In IPC-ranked competitions, to hand in any changes and subsequent attempts the coach or lifter gives the attempt card directly to a designated marshal (who should be a qualified referee). Both the coach and the marshal will co-sign to verify that they agree to the proposed change. This removes any ambiguity or misunderstandings when alterations are made. In IPF powerlifting the coach or lifter takes full responsibility for the attempt cards themselves and must personally give them directly to the jury table.

In IPC competitions the bar is increased in minimum 1kg increments; 0.5kg increments are only used for record attempts. For example, a lifter may go from a lift of 134kg to 136kg. In IPF powerlifting currently the bar can be increased by only 2.5kg (as 1kg increments are not permitted). Again, the 0.5kg discs are only used for record attempts. Hence an IPF lifter is likely to take the route of 135kg on the bar and, if successful, increase this to 137.5kg.

In IPC once the opening weights have been declared at the technical meeting (see Part 3: Competition) this weight can only be dropped by a maximum of 7kg, up to five minutes before the lifter's attempt. This prevents disruption to the order of lifting. To illustrate, lifter may declare an opening lift of 185kg, then five minutes before starting their first attempt, they drop the weight to 160kg. This would mean they would most likely need to be dropped from Group A into Group B, causing major challenges to the order of play for the LOC. Currently in IPF the weight can be reduced by more than 7kg, and in some federations there is no restriction.

While in IPF no long-legged suits are allowed, in IPC the lifter is allowed to wear a long-legged lifting suit, but they cannot wear a bench shirt or supporting lifting suit of any type. All the dimensions of the fabric and corresponding t-shirt should follow IPF powerlifting rules.

In IPC to execute the lift the lifter places their torso and legs in a prone position along the middle of the bench, as opposed to placing their feet on the floor (as in IPF). To make this accessible and safe for the athlete, the middle to lower section of the bench is wider than its IPF counterpart, measuring 61cm across, while the top section measures 30cm across. As in IPF powerlifting, the bench is 2.1m long. The bench stands no higher than 50cm.

The lifter is permitted to have extra strapping to help them stay on to the bench (see Fig. 2.30). If the lifter has a challenge with keeping their legs straight and prone on the bench due to their impairment they may ask to be assessed by a designated classifier. They may then be granted permission to position their legs differ-

ently (perhaps one leg raised and another flat on the bench). Any change must be reflected in their classification status.

While the IPC lifting platform is the same size as the IPF platform, it may have bevelled edges and access ramps where required. There will also be ramps for entry to and exit from the lifting area.

The minimum body weight categories for IPC lifters are lower than those for the IPF or non-disabled lifters, due to the different body compositions of, and add-ons for, amputee athletes. An amputee weighs in without their prosthetic device/s and is given an additional weight to their actual body weight to make up for the missing limb. For instance a single leg amputee (below knee) is given a 1kg increase to their actual body weight if they are in a category below 67.5kg. If they are in a weight class above 67.5kg the add-on awarded is 1.5kg. (See IPC Powerlifting rules and regulations for full body weight add-on per amputee grouping.) In all powerlifting the fundamental ratio of expressing the amount of

Extra strapping on the bench helps the lifter stay in position on the bench.

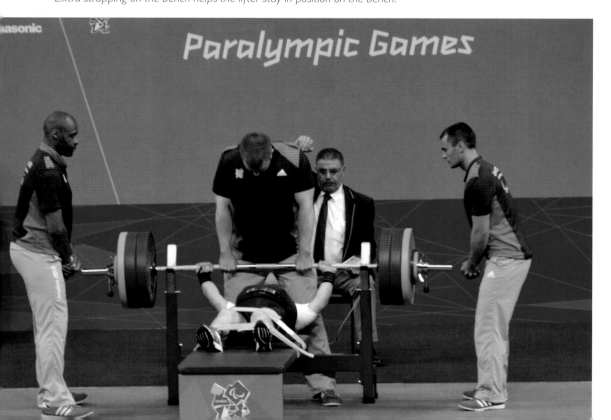

weight lifted vs the body weight of the lifter still stands.

The one rule that does not change across IPC and IPF is that when the lifter is about to commence their bench press they must not move from the elected body position once the start signal has been given by the chief referee.

IPF classification

The powerlifting classification system has been devised to assess Paralympic athletes in relation to their ability and impairment. The aim is to formulate an equal and fair system of competition for all who partake in each particular sporting discipline.

The nature of an athlete's impairment is medically assessed and scientifically measured to assess how it affects full functionality and the skill acquisition required for the sport. Each sport has a different system depending on the requirements and demands for that sport. For example, in powerlifting an athlete requires both arms and hands to be able to bench press. Alternatively, an athlete with an upper limb amputation could go on to become a world-class swimmer. Once an athlete has been successfully classified they are allocated a sports class status. IPC powerlifting is still primarily split into body weight groups in the same way as non-disabled powerlifting.

Athletes are deemed eligible to compete if their impairment fits into specific categories. These are physical disabilities as follows:

- Amputee, double or single, below or above knee.
- Spinal cord lesion and/or injury, spina bifida and polio.
- Cerebral palsy.
- Les autres ('others') which covers different impairments such achondroplasia (dwarfism) and locomotive disorders of the lower extremities.

To be eligible to compete in IPC powerlifting an athlete must be able to fully grip the bar without aids or prostheses. They must also be able to extend their arms with no more than a 20-degree loss of full extension on each elbow joint during a lift. Rules are likely to alter so it is important to keep up to date with all relevant information.

Once classified, each athlete is then grouped only by gender and body weight categories of the sport. In essence there are athletes with varying disabilities competing against one another. The sporting performance is measured, as all powerlifters whether male, female, non-disabled or disabled, on the strength to body weight ratio.

There is a complete IPC referee pathway, with associated referee qualifications, encompassing the elements of the disability experience. This includes working with large platform weigh-in scales, which are more suitable for wheelchair users. The referees continually attend seminars to help them prepare and set standards expected. (For further information contact the British Paralympic Association or IPC Powerlifting.)

Personal Equipment

As with any sport, it is important to choose the right personal equipment in order to train effectively and avoid injury. Each powerlifting federation has its own rules about the equipment that can be used in competition, and it should be noted that the IPF will only accept equipment that has been ratified by their Technical Committee. The simple rule is: check Federation requirements before buying any equipment.

When competing in the bench press the main items of personal equipment to consider are the lifting singlet, the lifting suit, the T-shirt, the bench shirt and wrist wraps.

Lifting singlet and suit

The powerlifting singlet is a one-piece suit with shoulder straps that covers the body from the thighs to the chest. All powerlifting federations require this to be worn in competition. An acceptable alternative is the lifting suit, which is a very tight-fitting version of the singlet and is designed to provide extra support. Again, different federations have different rules about the thickness of material and the measurements of hems and seams in singlets and suits, so it is a good idea to check the guidelines carefully. Failure to do so may result in a lift being disqualified. As noted before, within IPC rules Paralympic powerlifters are permitted to wear full-legged suits, whereas in IPF powerlifting the suits must be above the knee (see rules for specific leg length measurements).

Shirts

It is acceptable to compete in a T-shirt or a bench shirt, and there are specific competitions and lifting federations that have their own records and qualifying standards for each type of shirt. Whichever shirt is preferred, it must be worn under the singlet or lifting suit.

T-shirt

T-shirts should be made from plain cotton or polyester or a combination of the two and should not have any pockets, zips or features that could be deemed to assist the lifter in any way. It is advisable to check with the relevant powerlifting federation if there are specific rules about the size and type of any logos that may be used on the shirt and what may be considered as advertising.

Bench shirt

The bench shirt is a very tight shirt that helps to protect the pectoral muscles and the shoulders and is designed specifically to allow lifters to handle more weight. A bench shirt can add anything between 25kg and 75kg to a lifter's press so it is easy to understand its appeal. Nonetheless, the bench shirt is probably the most controversial piece of personal equipment in powerlifting as many people believe that it dilutes the true demonstration of raw power and, therefore, the essence of the sport itself.

Love them or hate them, bench press shirts have found their place in the sport so it would be remiss not to include them here. There are many available on the market and they vary according to both the type and thickness of material used in their manufacture and the type of fastening used on the back. They are available off-the-peg or, budget permitting, may be custom-made. There are a multitude of manufacturers and sponsors linked to bench shirts, and different federations have different rules so once again it is essential to check with the relevant organization before making a purchase.

It should be noted that Paralympic powerlifting currently does not permit the use of any type of bench shirt or top that does not constitute a plain cotton T-shirt. (See the IPC Federation rules and regulations.)

Material

At present there are essentially two types of material used in the manufacture of bench shirts: polyester and denim. Both fabrics are available in single-ply or double-ply, the latter increasing the weight a lifter can press and providing extra durability. It is also possible to buy canvas shirts but since these work in the same way as denim shirts, they are included in this category.

Polyester shirts are the standard shirt of choice for novices and world champions alike. The sleeves are cut on an angle, forcing the arms forward and preventing them from drifting back towards the face, thus increasing the weight that a lifter can press. Some shirts are made wholly from polyester while others use polyester for the front and a different material for the back. In addition, some are worn as a one-piece, some are completely open at the back while others have a split opening at the back that is fastened with Velcro. Denim and canvas shirts are similar in shape to their polyester counterparts but they support more weight and can be worn a little looser, making them much more comfortable. Generally, they have a split or open back which makes them easier to put on.

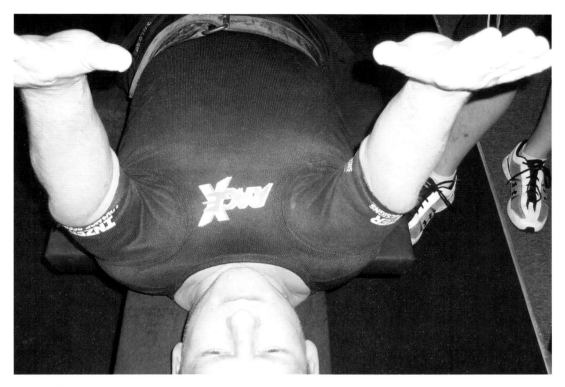

Bench shirt.

Choosing a bench shirt

As mentioned earlier, before choosing a bench shirt it is essential to check federation rules and guidelines because each governing body will have its own rules about which shirts are acceptable for use in competition. The hard fact is that any lifting records achieved at competition level will be invalid if the correct personal equipment was not worn when the attempt was made.

Different bench shirts have different characteristics and the benefits they provide vary accordingly. For example, closed back shirts work well for lifters who like to bench from the highest point of the chest, while open backed shirts are better suited to lifters who bring the bar down slightly lower on the chest, usually just below the pectoral muscles. While a lifter's shirt preference is linked to their lifting style, there is no choice about the fit as all bench shirts are designed to be very tight, especially under

the arms, and are not made for comfort. Quite simply, if the shirt does not hurt when the lifter brings the bar down to the chest, it is not providing sufficient support. Conversely, if it is possible to bring the bar down to the chest with ease, the shirt is too big.

Not surprisingly, the tight fit of a shirt makes it very difficult to put on, particularly if it is the closed back type which goes on over the head. For this reason, a lifter will require one or more helpers to ensure that all the seams are straight, especially those under the arms, and to smooth out any twists and wrinkles in the material. It is essential to ensure the shirt fits correctly since even a slightly twisted sleeve can skew the lift and affect results. It may take several minutes to help a lifter into their shirt so sufficient time should be factored into training sessions and competition warm-ups.

As is evident, several factors must be taken

into account when choosing a bench shirt, and all the available choices should be thoroughly researched before making a purchase. As with many things in life, the final decision is likely to be influenced by cost.

Working with the bench shirt

Having chosen a bench shirt, the lifter must now learn to work with it because the shirt changes the natural pathway of the bar, requiring the lifting technique to be adapted accordingly. From a biomechanical point of view, bench shirts are designed to resist the downward movement of the bar, and they change how the elbows and arms can rotate. To counteract this effect, many lifters find it helps to bring the bar to a point further down the chest during the descending phase of the lift, pausing at the level of the upper abdominals. Elongating the line of the bar's descent gives more time for the bar to reach the correct position before beginning the upward movement and consequently ensures the bar has enough height and breadth to bypass the lifter's face on the ascent phase of the lift. It can be imagined as a plane needing a longer runway in order to take off.

A bench shirt may cause considerable soreness under the arms until the lifter learns to adapt to it, so this should be factored into any training plan with sufficient time allowed to adjust. For many lifters, though, the additional weight that they are able to press when wearing a bench shirt makes all the discomfort and effort worthwhile.

Wrist wraps

Wrist wraps are designed to support the wrists and, as with bench shirts, they can be custom-made. They should be no longer than 1m and no wider than 8cm. Any loops or fastenings should be included in these measurements or the wraps will be classed as too long and will not be permitted in a competition. They can be shorter or narrower than this, however. As with so many aspects of personal equipment, the final choice of wrist wrap is largely a matter of personal preference established through trial and error.

CHAPTER 3

THE DEADLIFT

The deadlift is the last lift to be performed in any powerlifting competition and is the only lift of the three which begins with the weight on the floor. The lifter is able to choose when to commence the lift as there is no start signal to be granted by the chief referee. It is also set apart from the other two lifts by the fact that there is no momentum generated from any other force than the lifter to get the lift started. The lift is called the deadlift because the bar has no sway or give from the onset. Therefore, the combination of the bar and the weight is known as a dead weight. The deadlift is considered to be a true test of strength, mental toughness and sheer determination.

To commence the deadlift the lifter faces the audience with the weighted bar on the floor in line with their feet. They descend to the bar in a controlled manner and grip it tightly while maintaining the elected body position. Taking the strain of the weight, they draw the bar into the body, emit immense power and pull the weight upwards. The aim is to ensure that the bar travels in a vertical line until the lifter is standing fully erect with the bar motionless in their hands. Once standing upright and the chief referee is satisfied that the lift is complete, the lifter is given the command to place the bar back onto the floor. The lift should be performed while maintaining control of the weight at all times.

Three main deadlift styles have evolved: the narrow stance (also known as the traditional stance), semi-sumo stance and full sumo stance. The lifter's choice of stance will depend on their biomechanical levers, muscle adaptation and experience. For instance, a novice will usually start with a traditional stance since this is easier to learn.

The fundamental difference between the techniques lies in the positioning of the feet. For the narrow stance the feet should be hip width apart. For semi-sumo they are usually in line with the knurl markings on the lifting bar and/or approximately one and half times wider than shoulder width; some lifters will use the markings on the bar while others will use anatomical markers. For full sumo, the feet are placed as wide apart as the lifter's flexibility will allow, which may be as wide as the bar and discs, although the position of the feet should not pull the lifter's knees and hips out of line.

Performing the Deadlift

The three stances: narrow, sumo, semi-sumo

Narrow stance
The narrow stance is usually the first style taught to potential powerlifters. The lifter stands with their feet flat under the bar pointing forwards and hip width apart. They descend to the bar while keeping the back flat. Once the hips are lowered and in line with or behind the bent knees, and their hands can touch the bar, the lifter secures their chosen grip, maintains their back at a 45-degree angle and takes the weight by pulling upwards with the back and chest and pushing downwards through their feet. As the bar begins to move, the lifter continues to lead upwards via the chest until they are standing fully erect with the weight held at arm's length.

The key to narrow stance lies in the ability to hold the back firm and at least at 45 degrees throughout the lift. This requires a well-developed erector spinae, gluteus maximus, latissimus dorsi and trapezius, together with complete control of the lower lumbar region. To execute the technique well the lifter must draw the hips back then down, as if beginning to squat, keeping the back flat. This movement will bring the shins back from the bar slightly, making room for the top half of the body to come closer to the bar. From the side this looks similar to a long ruler that has been folded into three segments. The descent to the bar should be performed in a controlled, smooth movement.

Once the grip is secured the lifter takes the strain. The shins begin to move forward but do not become perpendicular with the ankles until the bar reaches just below knee level. At this point the hips draw towards the bar and the legs straighten. The back keeps pulling up and backwards to be in line with the bar. The full leg power does not come into play until the back has enabled the bar to move past the knees.

Sumo stance

The sumo style deadlift involves a very wide foot stance where the toes can be pointing forward or horizontally towards each end of the bar and anything in between. For some lifters the stance and foot placement are so wide that the toes can almost touch the weights. However, the actual leg span is dictated by the hip flexors and the lifter's leg length from the hips to the knee.

To reduce the distance of the pull this technique has a comparatively narrow hand grip, sitting just within shoulder width and between the knees. This style is best suited to athletes who have excellent power in the legs and gluteus muscles as the style dictates that the shoulders are forward of the bar, which prevents the back coming into play for the first quarter of the lift.

The aim of the deadlift is to pull the bar from the floor and stand erect. The sumo stance requires a far more vertical pull (from beginning to end) than the other stances. For the bar to follow the shortest path from A to B the back acts as a fulcrum and the lifter uses their body to create the best angled levers. In an ideal situation the shoulders would be forward of the bar, the hips and shins in a vertical plane, the feet flat and as wide as possible. This said, the stance should not be too wide for the knees, which would be indicated by the knees tending to turn inwards and the back being liable to fold.

Lifting sequence for sumo stance.

1
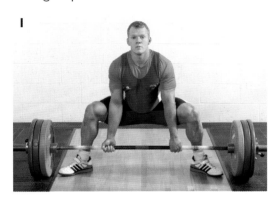

2
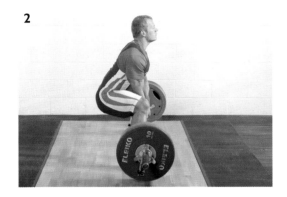

3

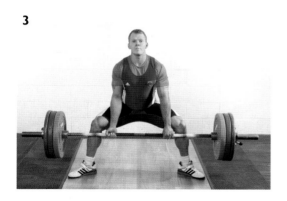

4

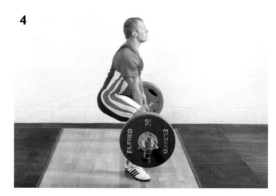

5

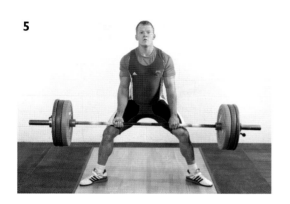

6

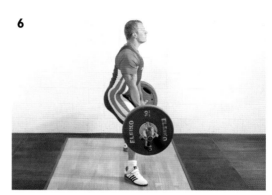

7

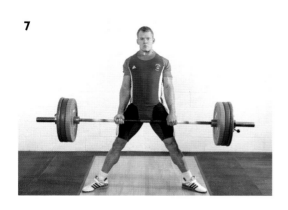

8

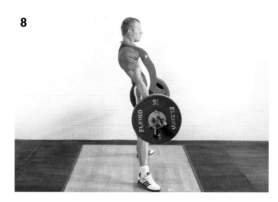

Semi-sumo stance

As the name suggests, this style's foot stance lies between the narrow and full sumo stances. The advantage here is that the lifter does have to pull the bar as far as with the narrow stance, so this works well for lifters who do not have the over-all flexibility in the hip flexors or the full gluteus power that is required for full sumo style. The semi-sumo style is often suited to an all-round lifter as it requires a combination of strength and flexibility, with the back and legs taking their fair share of the load. The pull is vertical compared to the narrow stance, and strong hamstrings, gluteal muscles and quadriceps are imperative. Accordingly, the lower lumbar region and the gluteals take a huge amount of the force until the bar is moving, while the legs are able to take more of the load and reduce some of the pressure on the back as the lift goes through the mid-range point.

Lifting sequence for semi-sumo stance.

1
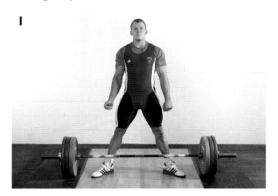

2
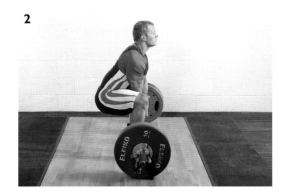

3
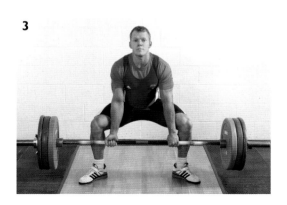

4
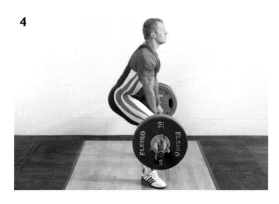

5
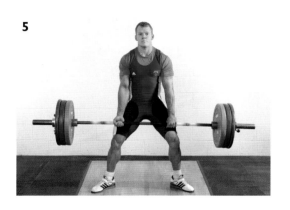

6
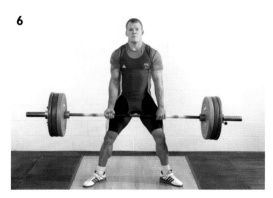

7

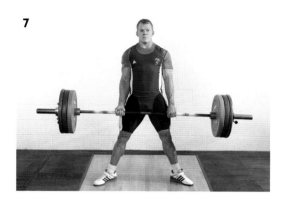

8

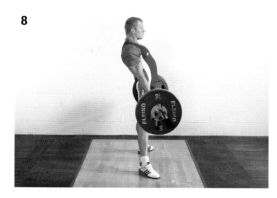

Grip

Grip strength and the ability to hold onto the bar are essential to completing the deadlift, since the pull of gravity continually drags the weight down towards the floor, forcing the grip to slacken. This becomes compounded as the bar itself has a tendency to rotate in the palm of the hands and also has some bend when the lifter begins the pull. The lifter's grip must counteract all of these variables.

There are three main styles of grip: the hook grip which is predominantly used for Olympic weightlifting, the alternate hand grip and the forward hand grip. The hand spacing alters according to the foot stance adopted. It is important to note when attempting to ascertain the optimal grip that the narrower the grip the less distance the bar will have to travel. However, the selected grip should not be too narrow for the lifter, which more often than not means less than shoulder width. A grip that is too narrow would drag the shoulders forward, in turn forcing the back to fight harder to remain in line. It should also be remembered that for all grips the fingers (including the thumb) should be, where possible, fully wrapped around the bar.

The hook grip takes the most time to master and can be very uncomfortable initially. To commence, the lifter should adopt the start position with their arms perpendicular to the bar and fingers spread wide but not touching the bar. The thumbs should be placed at an equal distance apart with the top segment around the bar. The first and second fingers should then be wrapped securely around the thumbs and the remaining fingers placed around the bar. This is a very secure grip but the thumbs can feel crushed, and for many powerlifters the discomfort can be a distraction, preventing them from concentrating on the actual lift. They often consider that it is not worth spending the time required to make the grip feel comfortable since it is only used for the deadlift and a few secondary exercises whereas, for weightlifters, this grip is the main anchor for the majority of their lifts.

The alternate grip is the most popular with powerlifters, because it stops the bar rolling out of the hands and is relatively easy to execute. Irrespective of the selected stance, the hands reach down to the bar, one hand goes forward and around the bar whilst the other rotates backwards and takes the alternate reverse grip. This is far more comfortable than the hook grip, although it should be noted that any grip will cause calluses to form on the hands as the lifter builds up their training load. While the alternate grip is extremely effective, it can restrict the shoulders and elbows by placing them in an asymmetrical position, resulting in extra strain on the joints.

The two hands forward grip is more favoured by bodybuilders or powerlifters who may have incurred previous injuries which restrict their flexibility. Here, both hands are wrapped forward

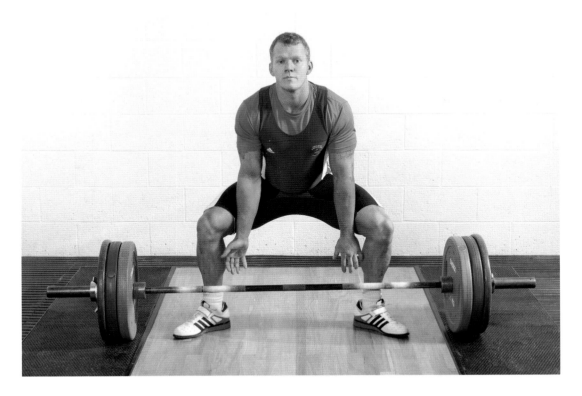

Alternate grip.

around the bar which can work perfectly well if the lifter has immensely strong fingers which are long enough to wrap around the bar. However, with this grip the bar will be pulled forward and pushed against the fingers which can make the lifter feel that the bar wants to roll out of their hands. They will therefore have to fight against any rotation of the bar throughout the lift.

Anatomy

As with the squat, the deadlift relies on three quarters of the posterior muscle chain and a quarter of the anterior chain. The difference between the two lifts anatomically is the angle of the pelvic tilt in relation to the placement of the spine and corresponding eye line.

Back

The back is the direct link between the hips and the shoulders and provides a pathway for the forces to travel between the lower and upper part of the body. It protects the internal organs and is the main carrying lever of the lift. Consequently, the most important thing is the ability for the lifter to hold the back flat and under no circumstances to fold too much in the middle. This requires flexibility, strength and a great deal of determination. (For a full anatomical consideration, see Chapter 1: The Squat.).

Hips

To enable the lifter to stand erect at the end of the deadlift, the optimal start position of the pelvis should simulate a quarter-squat and corresponding hip tilt. This creates the opti-

Deadlift body alignment.

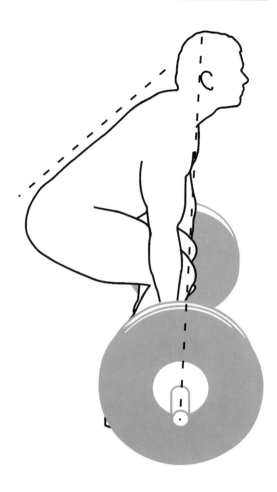

mal fulcrum and recruitment of muscle groups. The pelvic tilt, combined with the hips and extensors, plays a powerful role in bringing the skeleton into line, including the knees and ankles when locked. This avoids having to pull the bar around the knees, which is a very awkward movement.

If the hips are too high at the start of the lift there is a danger that the technique employed will become more akin to a stiff leg deadlift. This is a completely different exercise which, if used incorrectly, will put far too much torque force on the lower back and cause injury. It will also restrict the lifter as they attempt to complete the lift. On the other hand, if the hips are too low at the start of the lift the fulcrum and corresponding body shape will throw all of the resistance on to the quadriceps. This will make the ascent part of the lift more akin to coming up out of the bottom of a front squat, making the lift far more challenging. Unless the lifter is highly proficient at executing front squats they are very unlikely to complete the lift in this way.

Feet and ankles

The feet are key anchors in the deadlift, so it is essential that the lifter becomes aware of their feet and the role they play during the lift. The feet should be in full contact with the floor throughout the lift, and the lifter should almost be able to feel the texture of the floor through their deadlift slippers. The heels are the main pressure pad from where the lifter pushes and should be placed flat and perpendicular with the ankles. They should not be positioned so wide that they roll over or cause the ankles to twist or pull away from the heel. Whilst the heels are

perpendicular to the ankle, the toes are often splayed outward – more so for sumo deadlift, where they can be pointing towards the corresponding ends of the bar.

Since the feet create the base of the platform from which the lifter must push, any unintentional movement can cause the bar to sway and the lifter to lose control of it. For example, if the weight goes towards the toes, it is not anchored through the heel and dispersed throughout the foot, and the lifter will be pulled forward and the weight will be forced out of their hands.

With experience the lifter should be able to identify where best to place their feet, which includes understanding how the weight is disbursed across the foot at different stages of the lift. This will enable the lifter to utilize their feet to become good supports and stabilizers whilst generating a reliable platform from which to push. Eventually the lifter will be able to detect if they are losing control of the lift by how much contact their feet have with the floor.

In the long run it is better to practise the technique with a moderate to medium weight under the observation of a coach or training partner. Alternatively, lifts could be filmed or photos taken from various angles. This will provide feedback to the lifter and help them to increase their skill base until they are proficient enough to hold the body shape when under pressure. Such steps will help the lifter to lift better in competition and reduce the probability of incurring an injury.

Muscle combinations

When performing the deadlift the dominant muscle groups are the erector spinae, including the latissimus dorsi, rhomboid, trapezius and the gluteus maximus. The obliquus externus play a major role in supporting the back and holding the rib cage erect. Power from the lower half of the body comes from the legs, especially the hamstrings, utilizing the biceps femoris and semitendinosus, supported by the calves (gastrocnemius) and soleus.

Areas of vulnerability in the deadlift

The most common injuries linked to the deadlift are those of the back. More often than not these are caused by continually practising and reinforcing poor technique. In turn this leads to muscle imbalances so that there is a danger of becoming stronger in the wrong places, thereby reinforcing any weak links. For example, by continually training with a round back, the lifter will force the shoulders to take the load, so although the shoulders become stronger the back becomes weaker.

Back injuries predominantly fall into two main

THE DEADLIFT MOVEMENT

Descent

- Assume selected foot stance (start position).
- Contract shoulders and back.
- Release hips.
- Descend to the bar.
- Select grip.

Ascent

- Tighten quadriceps and gluteals.
- Grip bar tightly.
- Lift up sternum.
- Fire calves, back and shoulders.
- Begin to draw the hips forward.
- Use chest to lead the ascent.
- Spinae erector and lattimus dorsi hold the torso vertical.
- Activate trapezius muscles and tighten lower lumbar region.
- Use back as the main lever whilst working hamstrings and quads.
- Abdominals, including the obliquus externus, remain under tension throughout the lift.

categories: skeletal and/or soft tissue damage. For example, if the hip flexors are overly tight and the gluteus less developed than the lower back and legs, the pelvis can be pulled out of line, leading to groin strain. Alternatively, a weak lower back compared to very strong quadriceps and rhomboids can cause the lower back to fold under strain, again leading to displacement of the pelvis or muscle tears in the back.

Since you are only as strong as your weakest link, it is important to maintain an acute awareness of your muscle development and relative flexibility. If any weaknesses are apparent they should be worked into the training regime and the muscles systematically trained over time to do the job required for each lift.

It should be remembered that, for the deadlift, a lifter will require extremely well-developed back and legs. However, many injuries could be prevented if powerlifters paid more attention to their abdominals and inner core muscles, since a weak core offers little to no support for the back, which becomes increasingly fatigued as a competition progresses. Powerlifters are well known for putting hours of work into training their large powerful muscles and neglecting the smaller, less dynamic group of exercises, a trait which can and does lead to injury.

Developing Technique

The deadlift is the least technical lift of the three powerlifting lifts. Nonetheless, good technique will help the lifter to move more weight effectively and prevent injury. Throughout the lift the lifter should maintain an awareness of body posture and not allow the head to drop forward or the knees to travel too far inwards or outwards. If these misalignments are permitted too often, injuries could well occur.

Descent
As previously stated, the lift begins with the bar positioned on the floor in front of the athlete's feet. The feet should be hip width apart, or in line with the adopted stance, and positioned flat on the floor and under the bar. The lifter will need to develop an awareness of their feet to the point of almost being able to feel the texture of the floor through their deadlift slippers. This will enable them to identify where the feet are best positioned, including recognizing the line created between the heels and the toes. The pads of the feet will become the stabilizers from and through which the force will be pushed. Eventually the lifter will be able to detect if they are losing control of the lift by how much contact their feet have with the floor.

When the lifter is ready to descend to the bar a useful technique for creating and maintaining good form is to pick a point on the wall about 4cm above the eye line and to remember this spot. At the start of the descent the arms should be straight. The lifter should take a deep breath and, whilst contracting the upper back muscles, begin to descend to the bar, keeping their eye on the spot on the wall, which will tilt the chin up slightly. The knees should then be pulled wide (or pushed forward slightly if executing the narrow stance) and the hips pulled back and down. The hamstrings should be parallel to the floor. The hips should tilt down, arms should hang straight with palms open and fingers ready to grip the bar without the lifter needing to look down (this will take some practice).

The actual process of getting the hips into the final position varies slightly from lifter to lifter. Some lifters hold the hips static from the moment they tilt the pelvis down towards the bar. Others find it by rocking back and forth into it and, when they are ready to pull the weight, tilt the pelvis back slightly then thrust forward into position and pull as the hips come back in line.

Once the lifter has lowered themselves to the bar, assumed a quasi-squat position with arms outstretched, gripped the bar firmly while keeping feet flat and under the bar and is ready to take the weight, they will have achieved the start position. They may now begin the lift.

At this point the lifter should regain eye

contact with the same mental spot on the wall (if it has been lost in the set up-phase). This will keep the head up and help keep the back and chest up without tilting the head too far back or allowing it to drop too far forward.

Now the lifter should take the strain, elongate the back and bring the shoulders slightly in front of the bar, readjusting the hips if they are not in place. They should then tighten the grip, tighten the gluteus maximus and medius and begin to push the feet through the floor. At the same time they should start to pull the bar upwards, leading with the shoulders and keeping the hips down and not up and back.

The bar may now feel like a dead weight that won't move (hence the deadlift). It is at this point that a lifter will be tempted to break form simply to get the bar moving, usually by rounding and pulling through the back and not the legs. However, the focus should remain on pushing through the feet and pulling with the trapezius and upper back at the same time. This will activate the power generated by the legs and gluteals, and the bar will start to move away from the floor. The chin will naturally tilt upwards, helping to prevent the shoulders from becoming too rounded too early, and maintaining a flat back for longer – a huge advantage since this shortens the distance that the bar must be lifted.

Now the bar and shoulders rise in tandem. From a side view there is an imaginary line from the midpoint of the deltoid to the bar. As the bar goes through the first half of the pull the shoulders come back slightly and sit just behind the bar. Whilst pulling, the lifter must fight hard to stop the shoulders falling too far back behind the bar too quickly. Otherwise, they will become prone to falling backwards during the last quarter of the deadlift as they attempt to lock out the shoulders and knees.

Ascent

On the ascent the spine and hips together become a strong mechanism that moves like a well-oiled machine. As the chest takes the lead, the shoulders pull back (creating the full space needed to let the hips begin to pull through). It is here the gluteus muscles and lower lumbar region take a huge amount of the torque force as they as they become the cornerstone of the pivot.

Once the bar is moving, the lifter should keep it close to the shins while maintaining a flat back. When the bar is a quarter of the way up the shins they should begin to bring the hips forward to meet the bar. As the bar nears the knees, the hips must begin to pull back in line, aiming for an upright position.

With the bar just below the knees, the lifter can feel stuck if they have not drawn their knees back and out of the way. To keep the weight moving, therefore, the lifter must keep their hips drawing forward and the back moving up and back whilst trying to keep all the joints moving together. If they have managed to maintain a relatively flat back the bar will move slowly upwards. This is a good point at which to employ some good old-fashioned determination or, as sports scientists would say, mental toughness. The lifter must dig deep (both mentally and physically) as they are now three parts of the way there. They must hold form, not let the back curve or the shoulders slump forward and should use all the leg and gluteals power they can muster to guide the knees and hips towards one another. This will get the bar moving another few centimetres towards the last part of the pull.

In tandem with this the knees should be pulled back into a standing position. If the knees are unable to retract in time the lifter will have to lift the bar around the knees, making the lift much more challenging. At this point the lifter should remember to keep a tight grip on the bar and work hard to stop the fingers loosening off. They should continue to push the feet through the floor and keep pulling upwards throughout the entire lift.

If the back has concaved partway through (which is often the case) it can be very difficult to finish the lift. The more rounded the back becomes, the greater the challenge, and if the lifter cannot get the hips moving quickly enough they will not be able to get their hips to pull through.

At this stage the bar is halfway up the body, just above the knees. The gluteals become the dominant force and the lifter leads with the chest, which becomes the fulcrum, allowing the lifter to stand up.

For many this can be a particular sticking point so it is imperative to use the erector spinae by pushing up and back, use the abdominals by pushing them against the powerlifting belt and force all the power possible from the legs and gluteus to generate a major surge of power that will get the bar moving up another few inches.

By now the effort will be starting to show on the lifter's grip, and there will be a huge amount of torque force on the lower lumbar region and an immense strain on the quadriceps and hamstrings. The important thing here is not to give up since, as stated above, the lift is three parts complete. Therefore, the lifter should keep the momentum going by continually pulling and drawing the hips back into line, pushing the chest up and back, and pulling through the deltoids and trapezius.

To complete the lift the lifter must stand fully erect holding the bar at arm's length; the bar should not rest on the legs. This means that the knees should be fully locked out in line with the ankles. The pelvis should be perpendicular to the knees with no tilt. The shoulders should be pinned back and should avoid a shrug position. When the referee is satisfied that the lifter has finished and is standing fully erect they will grant the signal for the lifter to put the bar down. The lifter must keep their hands on the bar and maintain control of the weight as they lower it to the floor.

Getting stuck

In all styles of deadlift there comes a sticking point where the lifter feels as if the bar won't move or has got stuck. Good technique is essential to reduce this effect. As with all the powerlifting lifts the body acts as a fulcrum and axis to enable the lifter to move the weight. In the deadlift the hips are the operational fulcrum and the spine creates a weighted vertical line. This forms the main axis for the lift. However, as the spine is so long this does lead to a biomechanical disadvantage in the same way that the long seat of a seesaw could easily become unbalanced depending on the position of the pivot point and the distribution of weight.

The lifter can overcome this, either through genetic advantage, such as having a slightly shorter back with long arms, or they can build the relative muscle groups to counteract the long lever that the back constructs. For example, a very strong lower lumbar region and exceptional gluteus muscles will help the spine to hold static long enough for the hips to start tilting downwards towards the bar and shins. In turn this will help the hips to pull through as swiftly and as efficiently as possible.

The key is always to practise good form (shape of the body) and good technique. If the lifter allows the back to become rounded before the bar has passed the knees they will not have enough time to unravel the back and get the hips into a vertical plane before the bar reaches the mid thighs. This will produce a mechanical disadvantage and the lifter will feel stuck. If this happens the only way to get the bar moving again is to pull it around and over the knees. This will force the lifter to alter the pathway of the bar. In effect they will push the bar away from the vertical line which will result in a longer and more challenging pull.

If the lower lumbar region can stay strong and hold the torque force in a pivot position the lifter may be able to finish the lift utilizing their upper back and the trapezius muscles. The danger here is an increased likelihood of the bar resting on the thighs during the transition stage (a cause for disqualification of the lift).

Preparing to Lift

To perform a competition standard deadlift:

1. Stand behind the bar with it almost touching your shins and position your feet within your elected stance.
2. Descend to the bar whilst shaping your body into the start position. To do this pull back your shoulder blades, start to tighten your upper back muscles, activate the abdominals and begin to form a flat back, primarily by utilizing the rear deltoids. Start to tilt the pelvis slightly backwards. Keep the torso upright and descend in a controlled manner to the bar, leading with the hands which should be facing the correct way for the intended grip.
3. Take hold of the bar with straight arms, equal hand spacing and an extremely firm grip. Then take the strain and begin to pull. Note that, although the actual position of the legs will differ for each style, the method of pulling will be relatively similar.
4. Take a deep breath, begin to feel the weight, pull with the shoulders and chest and push through the feet. The bar will begin to move from the floor. As it does so start to draw the hips towards the bar and straighten the legs.
5. Keep the back from folding, bring the chest up and keep pulling with the shoulders. As you near the top of the lift begin to straighten the legs and work towards locking the knees and bringing the shoulders back.
6. Once the hips have been pulled back into line, the knees are locked and the shoulders are back, with the weight successfully held in the hands at arm's length, you must remain standing erect until the chief referee gives the command to lower the bar. This is given via the audible command 'Down' as the referee lowers their arm, demonstrating that they think the lift is completed. The bar can then be lowered to the floor.
7. You must lower the bar to the floor under control, which is achieved by slackening the back and leg muscles. When you have completed the lift and the bar is back in the starting position you should leave the platform and wait for the referee's decision as to whether the lift has been successful or not.

Sequence for traditional stance deadlift, front and side views.

1

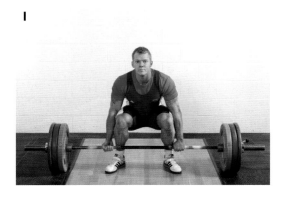

2

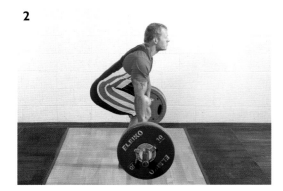

3

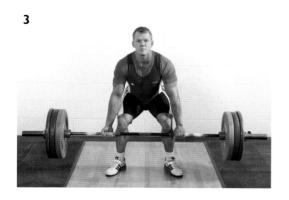

4

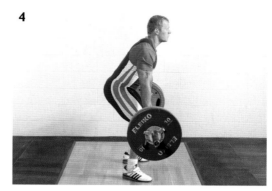

5

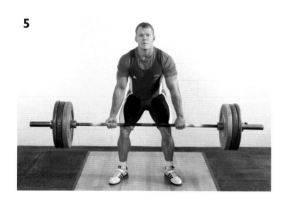

6

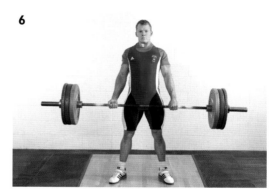

7

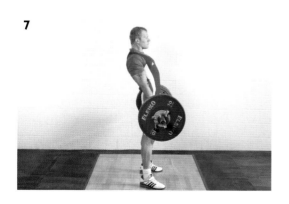

Personal Equipment

Deadlift suits
Many powerlifters are able to lift the same weight with or without a deadlift suit, although the suits do offer lumbar and hip support and can give the lifter confidence. Conversely, some lifters consider that the restriction within the groin and chest areas caused by wearing a suit is not worth the trade-off.

Deadlift suits are made from a similar fabric to squat suits but have a little less density within the woven ply. They are also cut slightly differently as they must allow the lifter freedom in the hip area as they move down to the bar. Like squat suits, they incorporate a harness system. This consists of strategically positioned – and very strong – seams around the hips and groin that work as an imaginary second set of ligaments. As sports science improves and understanding of the body develops, top manufacturers are continually re-designing their optimal suits. Therefore before purchasing a suit, a lifter would be wise to ask the different manufacturers for their latest suit specifications and seek their advice as to which suit would work best for them.

Erector shirts

Lifters often wear an erector shirt or tight-fitting shirt to perform the deadlift. Again, the drawback is a feeling of constriction in the chest area which must be considered alongside the benefit of back support. If a lifter decides not to wear a reinforced shirt that is permitted by the chosen lifting Federation, they must wear a plain t-shirt instead. This should not have any added seams or zips and should comply with the Federation's specifications.

Belts

A powerlifting belt is nearly always worn for the deadlift. Again this must adhere to the relevant Federation's rules and specifications. Lifters usually use the same belt for the deadlift as for the squat, although top lifters sometimes wear a softer belt for the deadlift.

Wrist wraps

Wrist wraps may be worn for the deadlift. These are designed to keep the forearms and wrists in a perpendicular line and help the lifter's fingers to stay wrapped around the bar. They must satisfy the same criteria and dimensions as the wrist wraps for all of the powerlifting lifts.

Knee wraps

Lifters can wear knee wraps, but not many do for the deadlift. Although they can help the lifter stand up more easily, their bulk makes it more difficult to pull the bar past the knees in a vertical line from the floor.

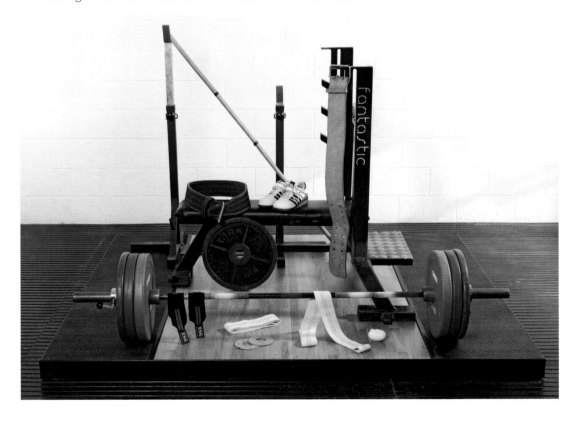

Starter kit for powerlifting.

Socks

Socks are worn long to protect the shins as the bar can cause abrasions when it is being pulled upwards.

Footwear

The closer the feet are to the floor, the less distance the bar has to travel so that more weight can be lifted. Deadlift slippers or shoes are thus flat, incompressible and create a sense in the lifter of having bare feet. The shoes should provide good support and have a non-slip sole; this is particularly important for sumo and semi-sumo stance because the lifter stands with legs wide apart, increasing the risk of losing balance and falling over.

Talcum powder

Talcum powder can be applied to the legs to help prevent the bar from slowing down or sticking on the thighs if it were to come into contact with the legs during the pulling phase of the lift.

Chalk

Chalk or resin can be applied to the hands to help the lifter maintain their grip on the bar during the lift.

All personal equipment may have the manufacturer's logos sewn or stamped on it. It is the lifter's responsibility to ensure that their attire conforms to the rules of the competition they have entered.

PART 2

TRAINING AND COACHING

CHAPTER 4

THE ROLE OF THE COACH

A coach creates the right conditions for the athlete/s they work with, encouraging them to look into themselves, identify their personal goals and the skills required to achieve them, and to learn, adapt and flourish. The coach builds a network of support and acts as guide and motivator as the athlete moves forward, sharing their ups and downs and moulding their dream into incremental goals so that it eventually becomes a reality.

All coaches at all levels must sieve through and assimilate information from a range of sources and then translate and disseminate the relevant components into a frame of reference that fits with each athlete's situation. These components can include anything from an athlete's physiotherapy report and competition history to the coach's interpretation of what stage the athlete is at, what they can deliver and which aspects of their training need work.

The coach must become a chameleon in the sense that they must absorb, learn, and adapt to the terminology of other disciplines; they must understand what terminology is required and acceptable at each coaching level; they must be able to use analogies and stories of the world to bring subjects alive and help athletes visualize what is possible; they must play different roles without losing their sense of identity; they must remain fully grounded in a sporting world that is complex, challenging and ever-changing. At the same time, they must deliver state-of-the-art information that is formulated through science, experience and in-depth knowledge of both the sport and the athlete. Just as important, the coach must be aware of the implications of anything they say, do and prescribe as well as their own behaviour because everything will be listened to, watched, monitored and referred to – a coach is always visible and accountable to other athletes, individuals and the governing bodies and agencies with whom they are associated. This intensifies the higher up the ladder they go.

To achieve all this, a coach must understand the context and key terms of each discipline they work with and be skilled in applying the relevant elements to their own area of operation. The delivery of their plan should be simple and varied with an element of fun. Above all, it should be underpinned by the ability to adapt and combine theory and learning, and apply this to the athlete in the form of a training programme that delivers results.

Personal Style

Each coach has their own style of learning and delivery. I begin by seeing a complete picture of the athlete in 3D. This means that when I watch an athlete perform a lift I can see the exact sequence of biomechanical movements that are creating the overall delivery of the exercise. In essence, I picture the finished article and all its moving parts. At times this vision is state-of-the-art in the sense that it is based on current 'real world' observations (as opposed to theoretical learning, which may be out of date), it questions what is seen and experienced in the here and now and it seeks to break down barriers by finding new ways to achieve goals and objectives.

To make this vision a reality I match what I am seeing to a blueprint in my mind of the perfect technical lift for that person. I then proceed to shape the appropriate technique for the individual. I am very aware of what I do not know and what is lacking in a lifter's performance so I continuously work to identify the missing links. I do this through research and by tracking down experts and having them design new pieces of equipment or provide knowledge to help in the quest of the perfect lift.

Let me explain this further. Imagine a priceless painting. The athlete is the canvas, and the dream and end goal is the finished masterpiece. I am able to see the individual dots of paint that make up the whole picture. To create the picture I add numbers to the dots and direct the order in which the dots should be applied to the canvass, in effect painting by numbers. Each athlete's goal and aspiration has the same number of components. It is the layering and ordering of the components on the canvas that differs.

The novice coach begins with the canvas, the numbers, the brushes and paints. As they progress they develop their own style and skills. Just like the athletes, they train and practise for years until they can replicate a masterpiece without the numbers.

Some top coaches may begin with the detail.

In this scenario they are able to mix the paints themselves, at times creating a formula never seen before. The detail builds and builds until the masterpiece evolves. World-class coaches move on to create a masterpiece for a global audience.

Responsibilities of the Coach

The core role of any coach is to guide an athlete through their sporting career; the ability to look after and safeguard the athlete is paramount. It is a multi-faceted role since the coach must serve as instructor, role model, mentor, facilitator, talent spotting officer, mediator, performance analyst, mentor, motivator, tutor and educator. To be truly effective, therefore, the coach must possess a wide-ranging skill set that includes elements of several disciplines.

The combinations of roles can be as varied as an individual coach's personality, strengths and weaknesses. On the other hand, all coaches perform a number of generic roles (first-aid provider, responsible adult, confidant, vital link to the relevant governing body, to name a few) and assume generic responsibilities which range from fostering a drug-free culture and promoting health and safety to ensuring all training sessions reflect the coaching code of ethics within the sport and are tailored to the individual athlete's needs.

The application of ethical conduct, procedures and guidelines for all involved when coaching takes place is the coach's moral obligation and, in most cases, their legal responsibility. Therefore, it is vital for any coach to keep abreast of all new regulations and guidelines. First and foremost this protects the athlete but it also provides a level of protection to the coach and the relevant sporting body.

The athlete/coach relationship
The coach/athlete relationship can be simple at times and complex at others. It should be founded on the concept of positive develop-

ment for both athlete and coach, and built upon trust and open, honest communication. In its simplest form the relationship works through a desire to achieve one goal which is to improve the athlete's sporting performance. The relationship can become complex because there is always a power imbalance which is in favour of the coach most of the time. This is because the coach has a big influence over selection and de-selection for events, so it is essential that the coach always works towards empowering the athlete. On the other hand, there can be times, especially if the athlete becomes very successful, when the athlete may hold the coach's reputation in their hands.

It is a working relationship that has an unwritten emotional contract between the two people involved. As we are human beings and thus prone to making mistakes, feeling vulnerable and, occasionally, being naive, there will always be times when the relationship may be open to exploitation, be it from the coach, the athlete or others. Therefore, from the very start, the coach must manage the athlete's expectations and set clear parameters for how the relationship will be navigated. For example, they must state upfront which data concerning the athlete they are able to keep confidential and which they are likely to share with outside agencies. There are stringent code of conduct contracts and procedures in place which will dictate this.

For a successful coach/athlete relationship to develop the coach should care about the person – the athlete they currently are, the athlete they aspire to be and the athlete they actually become.

Communication

To become a successful coach the ability to communicate effectively is essential, and most people have to work hard at developing this skill. A very important part of the equation is learning to listen, and the coach must be prepared to ask for honest feedback from others after delivering a message and/or instructions. Ambiguity can easily creep into the communication proc-

ess so clarity is essential and it should never be assumed that messages have been understood. This is the only way to create a reflective platform from which to work.

The coach should be sure in their own mind what meaning is attached to the message they want to communicate and be clear about intention and context. Where possible they should ask for the message they are communicating to be conveyed back to them to help ensure that all parties are clear on aims, objectives, any actions to be taken and who is to take responsibility for what.

Communication consists of both verbal discourse between two people as well as non-verbal communication, particularly body language, which can reveal a good deal about a person – a smile goes a long way. Silence can be used in a positive way during a conversation – for instance as an opportunity for reflection – so the temptation to try fill in the gaps should be avoided. It is important to give people time to think and to become comfortable in your presence, using humour where appropriate to help them relax. In all communications the aim is to make the exchange as open and honest as the situation will allow, in order to develop relationships and build teams that want to pull together.

Leadership and management skills

Leadership and management skills are essential to successful coaching. The key is to know when to manage and when to lead. A manager is precise and employs calculation systems and methods to achieve results. They excel at observation and replication. Managers are particularly good at looking for patterns in training diaries and using accurate methodology and statistical representation to predict performance output for individual athletes and for the sport as a whole. This helps to build a system based on tried-and-tested factors and, in turn, underpins and contributes to the body of evidence required by sponsors and governing bodies when funding is sought.

A leader, on the other hand, works from

the spirit within. They have a vision and believe everything is, or can be, connected to make that vision a reality. They have a deep respect for knowledge and education and combine this with an artistic, kaleidoscopic view of the world which enables them to link science, knowledge and experience in a fluid way and find ways to unpick things and put them back together in new combinations. They will go where others have not been, taking a calculated risk based on the laws of probability and a belief in the underpinning systems that can create instrumental change; a leader will lead change. Leaders challenge others to create new discourse and extend and break the boundaries of predetermined ideas. A leader continually creates and takes opportunities to become the best and lead a team to success. It is a leader you need when searching for state-of-the-art techniques and new ways for athletes and their sport to develop, grow and flourish in changing times and climates. A leader will find ways to become world beating and world leading.

Why coach?

The essence of coaching can be described as enabling an athlete to follow their true path. It is immensely joyful and satisfying to see others strive to achieve their goals, step by step, and fulfil their potential. This journey may take you, the athlete and others you work with down some unexpected avenues. As you progress,

---

JOB SPEC

What does it take to become a successful powerlifting coach? Among the many demands of the job a coach must:

- Understand and be able to coach a catalogue of exercises that underpin the squat, bench press and deadlift movements.
- Have a good foundation in the technical aspects of powerlifting such as conditioning, flexibility and muscle group activation that will aid performance output for competition.
- Be proficient in adding, loading and spotting the bar correctly within a training session (or coaching someone else to do this).
- Be able to produce an athlete-centred and sport-specific training programme.
- Be able to disseminate information in varying formats to match different individual learning styles.
- Understand the use of a training diary and related training principles.
- Be able to work with simple data (such as data from a training diary) and tailor it into an athlete-specific training programme.
- Have a strong understanding of the sport's governing body's rules, including knowing how and when record attempts can be made, the role of the technical officer (referee responsible for running a competition) and the processes to follow if an athlete does not make body weight.
- Have a good foundation in, and experience of, preparing for competition, to include the more intricate tactical elements such as reading and 'playing' the scoreboard and understanding the significance of lot order.
- Be able to deliver to and work with individuals from different social and cultural backgrounds.
- Be able to understand the coach/athlete relationship and how the dynamics can alter as the athlete's life changes; for example, if they get married the dynamics between coach and lifter change as a result.
- Possess good communication skills, including listening skills.
- Be prepared to learn and know when to hand over to others.
- Take responsibility for, and understand, any ramifications of their decisions and actions.
- Be honest with themselves and others.

you will feel and touch real emotion, good and bad, you will see the best of life; you will face many challenges and must choose whether to embrace them or walk away from them. Wherever you are on your journey, always be honest with yourself and with others and take something positive away from every experience.

A point often missed is that the coach's journey may not follow the expected path when setting out. On occasions, this may be due to external factors that cannot be controlled. I have experienced a talented athlete deciding that powerlifting was not their true sport, another opting to participate just for fun and another choosing to emigrate. All three could have represented Great Britain.

As a coach you learn at first hand the meaning of trust, commitment and respect. You build a deep understanding of people, cultures, what it is to be 'human' and, most importantly, what it is to be 'you'. All of your skills and beliefs will be tested and challenged over the years and you will have the opportunity to work on your continuing professional development and build transferable life skills. Along the way you will

stretch yourself and learn how to understand yourself better as a person and as an educator. You will learn how to acquire and share knowledge. You will develop the skill of listening and of knowing when to intervene and when not to. You will have the opportunity to become a small part of something bigger, for example by becoming part of your local sporting community or joining the national and international sporting community. Above all, you will have the opportunity to leave a legacy.

For all these reasons coaching can be a highly enjoyable and satisfying occupation.

A Generic Coaching Pathway

Coaches must build their own learning pathway in the same way that athletes do. Whatever the sport, all coach education programmes are structured incrementally and include a programme of theory, practice (coaching workshops) and observation. The exact learning components may vary slightly from sport to sport but, typically, student coaches enter at

Table I   A generic coaching pathway

Coach qualification	Athlete progress	Athlete needs	Coaching style	Sport specific coaching awards
Level 5	Elite Podium A-C funding band	Support/Sum of all below	Support	High performance
Level 4	High performance Development	Tactics International competition	Empower	International award
Level 3	Performance Talent confirmation National	Enhanced skill Service providers Athlete responsibility	Direct	National award
Level 2	Participation Talent identification Home countries	Technique Athlete specific	Coach	Certification award
Level 1	Introduction Regional	Familiarisation Basic skills Safety awareness	Teach	Foundation awards

Level 1 and progress upwards as far as they wish or their capabilities allow.

For those aspiring to become powerlifting coaches, good starting points for information and advice are British Weightlifting, the International Powerlifting Federation and, at elite level, UK Sport, the UK's High Performance Sports Agency (see Further Information). Local colleges may also be able to provide generic coaching programmes.

The following sets out a generic coaching pathway that is followed in various sports. For current sports-specific coaching pathways, it is recommended that you visit the websites of the relevant governing bodies.

Movement within the framework occurs both upwards and downwards, depending on the coach's progress in all the relevant components. The model takes into account both the athlete's and the coach's needs and outcome objectives at each development stage so that the relevant learning can be delivered.

It should be noted that all qualifications, coaching awards and content of any modules, seminars and workshops will vary and are the property of the federation/learning facility the coach chooses to go through.

Coaching education within powerlifting

Level 1

Coaches are taught all aspects of coaching safety. They learn basic training principles, including understanding strength training, machine and free weights. They learn how to teach an athlete to lift the bar safely and get it to travel along the correct pathway. This learning is supported by exploring joint movement and muscle and tendon actions, together with training in basic body alignment and the weight that an athlete at each level of attainment would be expected to lift. Coaches are also introduced to training programmes and learn how to interoperate them. They learn the rules of the sport, especially the body weight categories and rules for disqualification of a lift in competition.

Level 2

At this level coaches move to understand the more technical aspects of the three lifts. This is supported by kinesiology and basic biomechanical and physiological awareness. Learning should include simple ways to identify body composition. For example, if a lifter has a naturally wide stance, the coach may be able to establish through observation that they naturally have larger adductors.

In addition, coaches are introduced to recovery strategies, the corresponding methods of stretching and relevant auxiliary exercises. They learn to adapt warm-ups to the individual for training sessions and for competition. They gain an understanding of varying learning styles in order to make their training sessions more inclusive. They become familiar with session review strategies and learn how to deliver constructive feedback. They start to write basic training programmes (which would be checked by a mentor) and begin to understand where and how other professionals and service providers can contribute.

Coaches qualified at level 2 or above may work at any level up to and including their current level of qualification. For example, a level 3 coach is equipped to work with a range of athletes from beginner to talent confirmation level. Coaches are not equipped to work at a level above their existing qualification unless supervised by an appropriately qualified coach.

Level 3

At this level coaches are likely to be supporting athletes who are demonstrating potential for international competition. Thus, they need to increase their experience at a higher level. One way to do this is to attend official training camps and squads which enable lifters to train together and compete against one another. If this is not possible within the sphere of powerlifting, it would be worth contacting other sports. Experience of working with competition athletes is invaluable and generic lessons can be learnt across different sports, such as athletes' behaviours and the competencies expected from athletes and coaches in a world-class programme.

Level 3 coaches will be moving to more advanced academic theory and will have the opportunity to work with and learn from other coaches. They are privy to the enhanced technical methods that are taught to GB team members. They start to learn multi-disciplinary constructs such as physiology and recovery strategies and learn to develop more in-depth training programmes that introduce training aids, such as boards for the bench press and chains and bands for the squat and deadlift, to support the athlete's development through to European standard.

The athlete's training programmes become far more comprehensive and now consider the concept of progressive loading in other areas such as power and speed across different individual exercises as well as combinations of exercises. The coach learns about de-loading phases and what these might look like for different athletes. They develop a good understanding of the differences between male and female development and heavy body weight classes versus lighter body weight classes. They gain a solid understanding of record attempts and get to know who the main contenders are within individual lifts, within the sport and across the world. They increase their depth of knowledge in other areas, for example, psychological skills training and conditioning. At this level it is important the coach has a working understanding of how coaching instructions can be perceived and applied. They must come to understand the ramifications of the decisions and actions they put into place or are identified with. Sitting on the fence is not an option and the coach becomes accountable for performance output and results.

Level 4

At this level coaches learn to plot an athlete's performance pathway. They continue to work at the elite performance squads, with their success-ful athletes being selected for higher levels of competition. They gain multi-games experience, for example by attending competitions where athletics and powerlifting or non-disabled and disabled events run together.

Coaches are also introduced to the more complex, tactical elements of competition such as analyzing and 'playing' the scoreboard. They must study the rules to learn advanced strategies such as knowing when to move an athlete into a different body weight class in order to gain team points. They must also learn the appeals procedure, in particular when/when not to appeal, and study how appeals have been won in the past.

Overall, the Level 4 coach experiences a change of emphasis from participation in the sport to strategy and tactics but they must still be mindful of grassroots development. In other words, they must be able to work with the detail yet manage the big picture. They now begin to take up the mantle of a manager.

Level 5

At this level coaches are normally associated with world championships and the Olympics. More often than not, they hold, or have held, the position of National Coach, and the focus of their role moves from the individual to Team GB. They must now achieve the targets set by the sport's governing body and by sponsors. They coach other coaches as well as co-ordinate competitions, squads and camps.

Level 5 coaches are expected to understand athlete service agreements, write codes of conduct for athletes and coaches and create robust qualifying totals from entry level to podium level for their sport. They must work with others to ensure there is an effective pathway for athletes to progress from development to world-class and be able to create fast track programmes for athletes from other sports who might want to transfer into lifting. They are required to converse at board level (for example, to gain sign-off for equipment and funds for international training,

---

AREAS FOR DEVELOPMENT

These general developmental areas are applicable to all levels of coaching:

- Coaching ethics.
- Coach licence and registration.
- First aid.
- Health and safety when running training sessions, attending competitions, travelling and running squads.
- Insurance.
- DBS (Disclosure and Barring Service) clearance (formerly CRB).
- Safeguarding and protecting young adults and vulnerable adults.
- Inclusion, diversity and impairment.
- Exit strategies for athletes.
- Drug testing in sport.
- The role of the national governing bodies, including funding bodies and private funding options.

---

competitions and camps), they must understand business models and where stakeholders fit into the picture and be able to build relationships with different agencies. At this stage the coach's time is frequently divided between athletes, doctors, physiotherapists, service providers and lawyers. One minute they can be in a board meeting, the next discussing an appeals process for selection/de-selection, the next changing a light bulb in the gym. Adaptability is therefore essential and this level of coach is likely to be more of a leader than a manager. They continually strive to be the best they can be and to find ways to excel at the next level.

Top coaches complement their learning with courses, seminars and input from other disciplines such as business, other sports and peers (mentors) from 'high stake' backgrounds. An understanding of top level business is important because funding is involved and coaches must understand how to deliver results against budget. Mentors are also invaluable because, collectively, they provide the rounded perspective required to deliver at this level: I have a mentor from business, one from another sport and one who works for the United Nations. Together they have helped me to gain a better understanding of the human condition, develop the boardroom skills required to operate within a funded sports programme and consider in greater depth where sport is heading.

Training Programmes for Powerlifting

There are hundreds of coaching philosophies and epistemologies with corresponding methodologies that purport to underpin a successful powerlifting training programme. Each begins with a different viewpoint. Some are cultural while others are sports science based; many are built on the intuition, experience and observation gained over generations of coaching and lifting experience.

In the context of training programmes and helping athletes to become successful powerlifters, this book combines the scientific and statistical elements that underpin training loads with the physical and artistic elements that enable the athlete to create the optimal body shape to facilitate the correct pathway of the lifting bar. All the training templates given here begin with the athlete as a person, not just the level of attainment they have demonstrated at the onset. The main focus is on strength, power and technique while using weights. Special attention is paid to creating and maintaining body shape during the execution of the lift.

All prescriptive training programmes are progressive in nature. They can appear excellent when written down, whether as a statistical programme or as handwritten notes in a note pad. However, human beings very rarely fit into single categories, and once stress and emotion are added to the mix they become even less easy to categorize. Hence, it is always a challenge to get a methodology to align with human output. To help achieve this, all training programmes should be athlete-centred, taking into account lifestyle choices, include specific goals and targets and should be performed with excellent technique. This includes all stages of the warm-up section.

The training programme progresses in line with the athlete's development and performance so that, as each skill is mastered, another is added to the programme. The main difference between the various levels of a training programme is the number of sets and repetitions a lifter is able to achieve in a single training session and the number of sessions they are able to complete in one week.

All powerlifting training programmes aim to promote adaptation and learning, where adaptation is taken to mean that the mind and body adapt and evolve to accommodate increased tonnage in the sense of weight lifted. This modification of the human condition is brought about by exposing the mind and body to incremental physical and psychological loading, although the loading should go no further than the adaptive capabilities of the athlete.

Working at Different Levels

Learning should be a joint process for both coach and athlete. A training programme for a top level lifter is directed at achieving small, yet significant gains on the overall lifting total, for example, a 5kg to 7kg increase across the three lifts in competition. This can make the difference between winning a medal and placing fifth in a competition. The challenge of improving the total across the lifts becomes compounded as a lifter at this stage of their career is likely to have been training and competing for over ten years. As such, they will already have achieved their biggest strength gains, will have developed their overall lifting style, learnt how to focus and become able to prioritize their training sessions. Consequently, at this point the training syllabus has a different emphasis and the coach is analyzing small movements in great detail, an example being a pelvis tilt during a particular range of movement such as the last phase of the ascent in a squat. They are making greater use of expert and specialist knowledge from various scientific disciplines such as biomechanics, sports science and sports psychology (to name a few). All of this is sports-specific and athlete-centred with the aim of reducing the weak links that are hindering the athlete's performance and capitalizing on their strengths. This works in conjunction with trying to ascertain and unpick some of the underlying inhibitors to performance.

An intermediate powerlifter has learnt the basic techniques and thus focuses more on strength. Therefore, the aim of the training programme is to bring the lifter in line with some of their competitors and move towards international team selection. Accordingly, there is an emphasis on taking the technique to the next level and increasing exercises for specific muscle groups. At the same time the programme starts to consider other aspects such as electronically tracking the pathway of the bar, building extra conditioning sessions into the weekly regime and adding extra competition experience.

A training programme for a development level athlete focuses on teaching the three lifts. It works towards building muscle mass and strength and developing good muscle alignment so that the athlete can progress healthily in the sport. This type of programme includes many 'semi movements' designed to help the athlete learn the fundamental stages of the three lifts. It includes a variety of skill and strength

USING THE POLE TO FIND A NEW GRIP

The body is always adapting as a lifter develops muscle and improves their technique. Therefore the grip has to alter to suit their new body composition. To illustrate: bigger biceps require a wider grip. Here is an example of how the pole can be used to find a new/different grip on the bench press:

- Ask the lifter to stand up in the squat stance and hold the pole in front of them at arm's length.
- Get them to bring the pole to the chest while lifting the sternum and tightening the gluteus (as if waiting for the referee's start signal for the bench press)
- As the pole descends towards the chest, track the pattern of the elbows and observe if the grip alters at any point during the whole movement. (This is very useful when addressing an athlete's particular sticking point.)
- Having observed the pattern when the lifter is not under load you will be able to identify what needs fixing.

Full body warm-up sequence using pole simulating power clean.

1

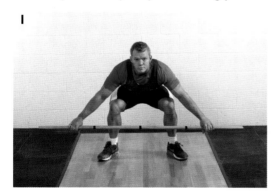

2

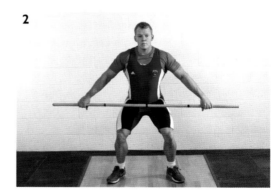

3

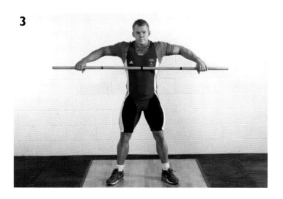

4

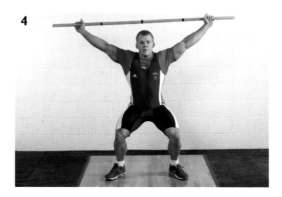

5

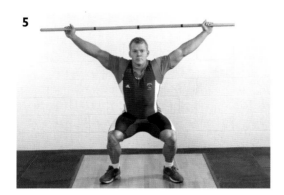

6

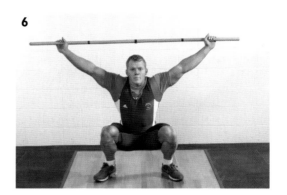

7

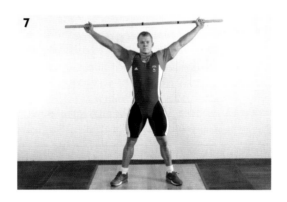

CHAPTER 5

COACHING IN PRACTICE

Prior to delivering a coaching session with a new athlete at any level a coach must gather a standard set of information about the individual, taking care not to omit anything. Below is the pathway I would follow.

Information about the Athlete

Profile
- Age.
- Gender.
- Previous sporting history.
- Previous coaching received.
- Previous service providers' inputs and outcomes (for example, if an athlete has received three years' input from a sports psychologist but has never managed to overcome their nerves).
- Medical history, including any physical restrictions or impairments which may hinder an athlete lifting safely and within the rules of powerlifting. It should be recorded if an athlete has an ongoing condition requiring medication that is on the banned substance list, in which case the situation would have to be managed by obtaining a Therapeutic Use Exemption (TUE) (see Chapter 10).
- Injury history, checking for repetitive injuries which could be intensified by heavy loading or by forming the body positions required for the three lifts.
- Preferred learning style and mode of personal contact between coach and athlete (for example, by text or phone call). Bear in mind that the mode of contact must be fit for purpose – given the confidential nature of certain communications, Facebook would not be appropriate! It is important that the coach maintains a footprint of all communications to athletes, service providers and other key stakeholders as, at times, it may be necessary to refer back to this.
- Time that can be given to training.
- Employment status.

Athlete assessment

Strength
Accepting that strength is a relative yet observable concept, within the context of powerlifting it is known as the demonstrative force when producing a competition 1RM (one repetition maximum) lift. There are many performance markers for this and it is advisable to choose a selection of exercises that will demonstrate upper and lower body strength without risking injury. An example might be simple sets and reps on a leg press machine, full movement bench press and quarter deadlifts, with the weight held in the racks (a set is a selected number of repetitions of an exercise performed as a group). The weights lifted and the lifter's ability to cope with the combinations of exercises can then be mapped to current lifters of a similar biomechanical make-up when they were at the same stage. If a lifter who has already been training within the specifics of powerlifting wishes to be placed on a fast-track programme, their full lifts can be filmed, their technique observed and the results compared to pre-set powerlifting qualifying standards.

Flexibility

The athlete's flexibility should be ascertained, especially within the hips and lower lumbar region, spine flexion, shoulders and ankles. This can be measured via a simple pole warm-up session and by asking the athlete to attempt a small circuit of exercises that replicate the movements required to complete the three power-lifting lifts (see physical assessment template below).

Psychological profiling

This includes motivation, confidence levels and the ability to focus and commit. These and many other components are measured by behavioural observation and standardized sport questionnaires.

Note that, when analyzing results, there will be issues that cannot be or will not have been factored in. As an example, a lifter attended a talent Identification Day that I was running. He was unable to complete the exercises and demonstrated very little strength. Yet his knowledge of the sport and enthusiasm suggested that he should have been able to perform better. As a coach I had to ask myself what I was not seeing; initially, I thought he may have a hip or lower back injury. The athlete returned a month later to retake the tests and went on to be placed amongst the top fifteen in the world. It turned out that just prior to the talent day he had undergone a vasectomy that he did not mention on the medical history and this had, not surprisingly, affected his performance.

Other factors such as anxiety or being in a strange environment can also cause the results to vary significantly. Consequently it is imperative to use your experience, knowledge and science to analyze what you are observing and question yourself before making an informed decision. Remember, an athlete's career potential could turn on your assessment. The athlete must have confidence in your decisions, so if you are unsure of something, talk to another coach at your level or preferably the level above. If in doubt organize two or three more training sessions and state clearly the aims and objectives of each session so you are able to manage the athlete's expectations.

Template for a physical assessment

The first time you meet an athlete/potential lifter, and prior to running a training session with them, you need to carry out a physical assessment. To do this:

1. Ask the individual to sit on a Swiss ball and return to a standing position. This may be performed for 3 × 10 reps, moving from a squat stance to an upright and balanced seated position. Observe the natural pathway the body takes during both the descent and ascent. Note if the hips move in one direction more than the other. Observe if the athlete is able to keep the shoulders back and chest up. Check the placement of their feet and note if the whole foot stays on the floor throughout the movement.

2. Coach the individual through 3 × 8 reps back squats using a pole (see above) to as low as is comfortable. Consider the alignment of the lower lumbar region, the natural depth to which the athlete descends and the speed and control of the movement. Meanwhile observe the flexibility of the shoulders as the athlete places the pole on their back. Do they take a breath during the movement?

3. Coach the individual through an overhead squat 3 × 6 reps, again using the pole. This is a squat with the hands above the head whilst the elbows are in line with the ears, holding a pole or bar. Note if the lifter is unable to get their arms high enough as this may be difficult for lifters of larger build with muscle mass on their shoulders and chest. Consider where the arms sit when they are over the head and the hips begin to descend. Do they stay in line with the ears or do they dramatically move forward or backwards?

4. Leg press machine 3 × 6–8 reps. Do the feet stay on the pressing plate? How far is the individual able to bring the machine down?

If this is challenging it could be due to very tight Achilles or hamstrings which means the athlete will find it difficult to perform a full squat. You will therefore need to design a training stage (possibly two) that focuses on improving flexibility in these areas.

5. Talk the athlete through the bench press movement, 3 × 8. Meanwhile observe how they position their arms in line with the pole whilst it is held at arm's length. Do all of the fingers go around the pole, including the thumb? Do the wrists roll back as the pole begins to descend? When the pole travels does it move towards the athlete's chin or does it tend to drift towards the abdomen? (Note that the optimal line would be in the middle of these two points.) Do the shoulders remain on the bench?

6. Ask the individual to sit in the centre of the Swiss ball and instruct them through a very light band or dumbbell shoulder press. Observe the shoulders, back and elbows and how they stay in alignment; 3 × 6 to 8 reps should be sufficient for this.

(Note that the resistance and sets and repetitions will vary according to the athlete's previous sporting history.)

In summary the assessment template would read as follows:

Squatting to Swiss ball/resting momentarily standing up	3 × 10
Back squat	3 × 8
Overhead squat	3 × 6
Leg press	3 × 6–8
Bench press	3 × 8
Dumbbell shoulder press	3 × 6–8

It is important to remember that when you analyze the assessment results you will be comparing them to a set of criteria. Therefore, if they do not come up to the required level, you will need to manage the athlete's expectations accordingly, and without knocking their self-esteem. If they are not best suited to powerlifting, be prepared to offer them alternatives such as a different sport, coaching or refereeing.

If you are satisfied with the results of this assessment, you are ready to deliver a training session.

Organizing the Sessions

As you progress you will design your own format, although it should be remembered that there will always be specific elements that you cannot leave out of your training sessions, for example health and safety.

Guidelines for successful coaching sessions

For anyone new to coaching, the following is a good general guideline of how to proceed.

- Share the intended format, aims and objectives of the session with all concerned.
- Advise lifters of any changes in the proposed programme or aims of the training session.
- Clearly demonstrate how the session will meet the athlete's training needs and their personal coach's objectives and how it will align with the athlete's performance goals.
- Provide diversity, promote interest and challenge the athlete mentally and physically.
- Make sure each lifter is given the opportunity to demonstrate a strength and to work on weaker points.
- Allow for individual differences.
- Provide constructive and positive feedback, both during and after sessions, for example via email or by sending footage of training sessions, sharing coaching tips with the athlete's personal coach or with the athlete direct.
- Adapt to your environment – you may not always have access to the equipment you would like and will need to think on your feet and refocus training sessions accordingly in order to deliver what is needed.

Sets and reps for powerlifting

Training programmes prescribe the intensity and load to be undertaken at each training session in the most energy-efficient manner possible. They create progressive loading phases that are entirely manipulated by conscious muscular activity. The level of intensity suggested for an athlete's training session is usually derived from a percentage of the competition 1RM (1 rep maximum) lifts already achieved. It should be noted that various factors can affect muscle power output, such as the angles of the joints or levels of dehydration, and that one programme does not suit every lifter. The training components to choose from will be the same, but the order and intensity of each will always vary according to the athlete's strengths and weakness that are to be worked on.

A formula for progressive loading

Over a period of thirty years of travelling around the world as an athlete, referee and coach I have developed this formula, incorporating many cultural views gathered along the way. During this time I have listened to, talked to and observed countless athletes and coaches on every continent at every kind of venue – from world championship events, with over 200 countries competing on one platform, to local back street gyms.

Sets and reps are well suited to the three fundamental powerlifting lifts: the squat, bench press and deadlift. Here I explain how to put sets and reps together to build the basis of a training plan. I have developed this formula from years of travelling the world as an athlete, referee and coach and incorporating many cultural views. During this time I have talked to and observed countless athletes and coaches at venues ranging from world championhip events to local gyms. The following would be a good start point for an intermediate athlete, noting there may be other components that an individual coach would want to include:

Warm-up as appropriate to undertake 85 per cent of previous 1RM. To illustrate, the athlete may be able to lift a top weight of 100kg (their Personal Best or PB) so 85 per cent would be 85kg. They would therefore warm up to 85kg. It should be noted that warm-ups are not counted in work sets.

Aim: 5 sets × 5 reps at 85 per cent with 90 seconds rest between each set.

Each group of five constitutes the whole exercise or objective.

When the athlete becomes competent at the above, begin to reduce the rest time, for example: sixty seconds rest, then thirty seconds rest, all at 85 per cent.

When five sets of five can be performed well, it is time to increase the weight and move to four sets of four and so on – see the formula below. For some athletes this may take two weeks, for others it may take four. As with many things in life, it is quality that counts, not quantity. It is important to know your athlete. If you think they may struggle at a particular point, start off slightly lighter and build in the necessary time to complete.

PROGRESSIVE LOADING FORMULA

A formula for progressive intensity aimed at producing a 1RM lifted:

4 × 4 at 90% (90kg) with 90 seconds rest, then 60 seconds rest, then 30 seconds.
Followed by:
3 × 3 at 95% (95kg) with 60 seconds rest, then 30 seconds rest.
2 × 2 at 100% of previous PB (100kg) with 60 seconds rest, then 30 seconds rest.
1 × 1 × 1 at 110% (this is equal to two competition lifts at 110kg) with 60 seconds rest. This equals two times 110% – 10% above current PB.

Devil sets

Top level coaches will use a variety of formulae and technique-specific exercises to promote muscle adaptation and strength. Here is a bench press specialist exercise which I adapted and which has been used by world-class bench pressers. (They are called devil sets because this exercise is very challenging and is predominantly based around three sixes.)

This exercise helps to promote stability under load and increase concentration levels when a lifter is being physically challenged, thereby warranting a lighter weight: between 45 per cent and 60 per cent of maximum 1RM for each grip. Each set is continuous with no rests between the change of grip.

Perform six sets as set out below:

	1 × 6 wide grip
Set 1:	1 × 6 medium grip
	1 × 6 narrow grip

18 reps = 1 set. Rest accordingly between each set.

It should be noted that each lifter will have a Personal Best (PB) on every exercise undertaken. As each training cycle begins, the weights are moved to the next denomination. This may well involve the use of a resistance band if an extra disc on the bar is too much of a jump. As body composition and strength alter across muscle groups, a lifter could well be on 4 × 4 for one group of exercises yet be on 2 × 2 for another.

Taper phase (decreasing volume, increasing intensity)

To produce a 1RM within powerlifting a lifter must decrease reps and increase the weight lifted. The training regime should manipulate the training so that top performance output can be produced at exactly the right time. If a lifter stops training they lose strength and training effects such as flexibility. On the other hand, if they push too hard they become fatigued. Either way, they cannot perform to their best. The nature of the sport and the need to continually push for adaptation means there is always a risk of over-training and fatigue setting in. To

counteract this, the training programme should include a taper phase in the final stages. The traditional approach to this is to decrease the reps and overall volume of training and increase the weights to be lifted as the competition date approaches.

In powerlifting there is a taper phase both within the daily training programme and the content and number of sessions per week as the lifter approaches their lifting goal. For some lifters this may mean taking a complete rest for between two and five days before a competition. For the majority of lifters this continues to a rest phase post-competition. The number of rest days and the activity undertaken (for example, light stretching, pole work, massage or physiotherapy), will be determined by the athlete and the coach.

The above working model is not always obvious to some. To illustrate, over the years many individuals have come to me convinced that they are more than capable of a credible powerlifting squat 1RM based on their being able to achieve, for example, 15 reps of 120kg. Theoretically, this is equal to a 1RM of 140kg so they think this is what they can achieve. However, the reality is that if you train for reps you will become an expert at producing reps. In my experience it is highly likely that, at best, the athlete will produce a 1RM at 130 kg. This is because the extra weight tends to throw the lifter forward on the descent and bring their hips up too early on the ascent with the result that they do not break parallel and fail the lift within the powerlifting rules.

Recovery

Fatigue can be defined as a temporary imbalance between training and recovery. Recovery from a training session is a key component of successful adaptation and strength building. A coach must look for and observe signs of fatigue in their athlete at all times, for example increased susceptibility to colds, increased irritability or reduced performance on two or three consecutive training sessions.

By the very nature of the sport, athletes

continually strive to lift heavier and heavier weights and it is often seen as a weakness to have a deloading phase (fewer weights and increased volume). Often it is the lifter who wants to continue lifting heavier weights in a bid to impress the coach. However, rest is critical and it is far better to take a few days' complete rest post-competition or after a heavy lifting phase. There are many ways to enhance recovery such as targeted physiotherapy sessions, psychological training, heat treatment, massage, and good quality (deep) sleep. However, I cannot advocate enough the importance of putting into place a deloading phase within any athlete's training regime.

Stages of Development

The traditional pathway of general strength programmes across the three powerlifting lifts follows a pattern of:

5 reps × 5 sets
4 reps × 4 sets
3 reps × 3 sets
2 reps × 2 sets
1RM

This formula will work adequately for the first two years of training. If a lifter shows potential to become a champion within the sport I suggest the following training recipe:

Level: Novice – Talent
The lifter should be proficient in the following technical aspects of the three lifts:

Squat
- Find foot stance without looking down at the floor.
- Ascertain where the bar sits on the back.

Bench Press
- Learn to find the highest point on the chest when lying down.

- Learn to press from the latissimus dorsi and not through the front deltoids.

Deadlift
- Keep the back flat and chest up during the execution of the lift.
- Ascertain the optimal grip and foot stance.

In addition, they should:

- Understand the rules for failing a lift during competition.
- Be aware of drug testing procedures.
- Understand the process of a competition including kit check and giving in first-attempt cards.
- Know how to manage 'dead time' at competitions (the time between the weigh-in and the first lift and between lifts).
- Understand the importance of athlete responsibility, particularly as it applies to the training diary which must be truthfully completed in order in order to achieve predicted results.

Level: Intermediate (British champion and above)
The lifter should be proficient in all of these Novice-level points plus:

- Employ simple goal-setting.
- Begin to become independent/self-sufficient, for example being able to listen out for the referee's signals during a competition and not depend on the coach for instructions.
- Understand the role of nutrition in relation to competition, for example when and what to eat in relation to weigh-in times and to actually lifting.
- Acquire their own lifting attire (previously they may have borrowed it).
- Begin to employ psychological skills training.

If the athlete lifts to the required qualifying standards they will come under the tutelage of a performance coach who will build upon the attributes and technique they have already established.

The coach will look to increase consistency and power within the muscle groups as they cross over during the execution of a lift, for example transference from the biceps to the triceps as the weight travels from the mid range to the upper quartile during the ascent phase of the bench press. This can be measured by the speed of the bar during the lift (see Chapter 2). To facilitate this, the coach will introduce the athlete to holding a maximum weight under control whilst maintaining the elected body shape throughout the duration of the lift, be it full or part movement. The maximum weight should be outside the confinements of the lifter's current 1RM and close to their failure point without causing distress or injury. For example, if the lifter's competition 1RM squat is 200kg the coach would be looking for them to perform a quarter squat at 220kg. In this situation they are not producing the full movement but they are now pushing the boundaries of weight lifted.

This approach enables the coach to identify weak links within body composition, alignment and body shape and to change the training regime accordingly. Hence, training begins to include the time spent handling the maximum load and the time holding the body shape and exercises to increase concentration span. At times, the lifter is under immense load so the coach's input is vital here.

The coach now employs a more scientific approach, measuring the actual speed at which the bar travels and tracking the pathway the bar takes during the execution of the lift. In tandem, they also monitor and continually evaluate the combination of exercises, changes in power output and the athlete's body composition.

Psychological skills training now becomes more athlete-specific, often concentrating on how to compete and cope with long training cycles. The use of training diaries becomes imperative as more complex data begins to be recorded (see Chapter 6). This keeps lines of communication open between the athlete and their personal coach and between the performance coach and the personal coach.

Level: International

The biggest difference between national and international events is that the athlete and coach are now representing their country, not themselves or their club. At these competitions it is the head coach who chooses the weights to be lifted and not the athlete. In some ways this can take the pressure off the athlete as the coach takes full responsibility for the team's final performance output. However, athlete responsibility is key as they must still deliver the performance.

The coach is now looking to improve power output, control and consistency throughout the lift. The athlete now progresses to lifting more weight, more often with far more technical detail. This requires full focus and a range of support services. To illustrate, where the athlete was previously lifting 1 × 3 at 220kg in a quarter squat movement, they would now be expected to begin this phase by completing 3 × 3 of at least 220kg, then moving up to 5 × 5 within the same weight range. They would then be expected to do a further two heavy powerlifting exercises followed by two secondary supportive exercises.

By now pre-competition strategies are becoming more important. For example, three weeks before competition all the strategies should be in place such as visa and passport arrangements, acclimatization phases, what and when the athlete will eat, their source of fluids (in relation to drug testing), travel to the competition venue, who will coach them on the day (including in the warm-up room and stretching phases). This is a joint responsibility of the athlete, the coach and team manager. Nobody should presume that a third party is taking care of these.

By this point the athlete should have built up quite a stock of lifting kit including lifting suits, a belt, correct shoes, chalk and water bottles, which they must bring to training sessions.

They need to compare their own performance with that of the opposition and ask themselves honestly if they are really putting in as much effort as a lifter from another country and another continent. This is a real turning point and the coach is there to encourage and support.

Some lifters go on for years at international level while managing a balanced lifestyle. Others will push to go still further.

Level: World class

The key difference between an international and a world-class powerlifter (besides the athlete's genetic propensity and their previous training) is having the time and funds to commit to being a full-time athlete and putting powerlifting at the forefront of their lives. It is worth noting that, although powerlifting is not an Olympic sport and therefore not automatically subject to funding, there are exceptional powerlifters who have obtained world level medals and records without any financial support.

A world-class lifter carries out all of the activities outlined above, but their performance is now analyzed from a range of perspectives including sports science, nutrition, performance lifestyle, medical, psychological and physiotherapy. These are full scale interventions, designed and delivered according to the athlete's performance needs. At this stage it is all about performance output and much less about the person.

If the athlete chooses to accept funding or become sponsored, the bottom line is that the investor will seek a return on their investment. At this level the athlete is only judged on medal achievements: no medal, no funding. The funding enables the individual to become a full-time athlete. Accordingly, they are able to undertake training up to three times a day, seven days a week. Two of the three days could include recovery and pre-habilitation sessions, as well as lifting weights.

A funded athlete is supported financially through the whole process and may be bought out of their employment for the period of their funding. This is no easy option and needs to be very carefully considered from a range of perspectives (family, lifestyle and career, as these must all be put on hold), noting that world class lifters are now lifting up to four times their body weight and the required commitment is absolute.

Formula for a Competition Training Programme

The following formula is based on my coaching experience and on working alongside and observing other esteemed coaches from across the world. It is the approach I take today, although it is also a work in progress. It has created champions, and it has also served as a platform for building transferrable skills that have helped individuals succeed in other areas of their life.

All training programmes are progressive. All numbers and percentages used to create the programmes (the 'ingredients') are the same. It is the combination of numbers, percentages and exercises and their execution that make the difference between success and failure. It is not the 'what' that matters, it is the 'how'.

Preparation

Start point and goal

Identify what you know about the athlete as a person – for example, are they lifting for themselves, for others, to improve their self-esteem or for the sheer love of the sport? There is no right or wrong answer here but it is critical for you as a coach to know your starting point. Identify the lifting goal – for example to lift 120kg at a body weight of 60kg in fourteen weeks' time.

The time factor

Work out how many weeks there are available to work with, for example twelve weeks to the British championships. Split the weeks into two parts, A and B, each being six weeks if twelve full training weeks are available. Alternatively, choose one longer programme with built-in assessments along the way. This would most likely suit a ten-week training cycle.

Impediments

Identify the weak links that will make it more difficult for the lifter to achieve their goal, for instance overly tight hamstrings or difficulty in maintaining body weight. List these in order of importance (you cannot fix everything in one go).

The venues

Consider where the lifter will be training through-out the training cycle – it may not always be their local gym. Remember each gym will have different equipment, coaches and loaders available so this needs to be factored in. Match the exercise to the weak body part and the gym in which the lifter will train. For example, to exercise the back muscles in one gym the lifter may have to use machines rather than free weights, while in another gym you may need to prescribe prone rows with dumbbells as opposed to a bar. In other words, change the exercise according to the environment and the muscle group.

Creating the programme

Once you have ascertained the days of the week when the athlete is available to train and have compared this to their workload in their daily life, you can begin to plan individual training sessions, for example heavier days and lighter days. Accordingly, you can choose the exercises that are most important and prioritize them according to the weak links, body composition and ultimate lifting goals. Many athletes train on Monday, Wednesday, Friday and Sunday (this frequency works well for any days of the week as long as you employ recovery strategies).

Think about what the lifter's Personal Best is in all exercises and how far they can progress in the time you have available. All exercises should be progressive and this can be achieved by simply adding two extra reps over four weeks, or adding a 500g disc. Work out where the athlete needs to up-skill, for example performing part movements, new exercises and achieving different body shape under load.

The exercises

You are now at the point of working out the main powerlifting exercises. If your first main powerlifting exercise is for a 1RM at 80kg for the bench press a way forward would be:

Week 1: 5 reps × 5 sets at 60kg
Week 2: 5 reps × 5 sets at 62.5kg
Week 3: 4 reps × 4 sets at 65kg
Week 4: 4 reps × 4 sets at 67.5kg
Week 5: 3 reps × 2 sets at 70kg
Week 6: 2 reps × 2 sets at 72.5kg
Week 7: 2 reps × 2 sets at 75kg
Week 8: 2 reps × 1 set at 77.5kg

Now build in two secondary exercises beneath the main exercises for each of the main training days, for example dumbbell bench press. For elite athletes you can go up to three big powerlifting exercises and two secondary types of exercise (such as light resistance for shoulders) in one training session.

Only prescribe exercises that the lifter can perform proficiently by themselves or with their personal coach. Keep advanced exercises for training camps and one-to-one coaching sessions.

TRAINING PROGRAMME – CASE STUDY

The following is a real life scenario of an athlete that I coached for six years.

Athlete profile

- Female.
- 20 years old (this is classed as a junior lifter within powerlifting).
- Two years' training and competing within powerlifting, performing all three lifts.
- One year competing in bench press only competitions.

- Intermediate national standard within powerlifting.
- Athlete lifts in both unequipped and equipped competitions.
- Previous sporting history: international level as a junior and at national level as a senior in athletics within the discipline of shot put.
- Athlete has previously worked with a sports psychologist concentrating on competition anxiety.

Ongoing technical issues
(This is a record of the lifter's technical issues that resulted in red lights and failed lifts within competition to date.)

- The bar tended to roll down the lifter's back during the descent of the squat.
- The lifter tended to change elected body movement during the bench press, moving their feet off the floor.
- The lifter shrugged the bar at the completion of the deadlift (causing downward movement of the bar and resulting in failure of the lift).

Performance output challenges
- Over anxiety pre- and during competition.
- Losing too much body weight pre-competition, which has caused a negative effect on body composition and a subsequent loss of strength. To begin with, the lifter had a low body mass index (BMI) and during the last stages of preparation had lost up to 2kg pre-competition.

Aim of the next sixteen weeks training blocks
- To obtain an overall lifting total of 347.5 kg in the Under 48kg class at the British unequipped championships, which would increase the lifter's previous total by 10kg.
- To close the gap between the weight lifted in the gym and at competitions.
- To improve the total amount of lifts gained on platform (on average five out of a possible nine lifts are gained), which has a direct

correlation with the lifter's enhanced competition anxiety and inability to maintain body shape during the lifts.
- To improve the following PBs.

Squat 117.5kg (PB on competition platform: 115kg; PB in the gym: 125kg.) This would be an increase of 2.5kg during competition, thus reducing the gap between gym and platform lifts from 10kg to 7.5kg.

Bench press 75kg (previous PB on platform: 70kg; 75kg in the gym). This would be an increase of 5kg during competition, thus closing the gap between competition and gym lifts – a much sought after position to be in.

Deadlift 155kg (previous PB on platform: 152.5kg; 152.5kg in the gym). This would be an increase of 2.5kg during competition and, for the first time in the lifter's career the competition lift would exceed a gym lift, which at this stage of lifting could be taken as an indication of the lifter's potential to become a champion.

*Breakdown of the following
16-week blocks of training:*
Phase 1. Four days complete rest, ten days de-load phase = two week block
Phase 2. Two weeks
Phase 3. Four weeks
Phase 4. Eight weeks

The length of each phase is dictated by the lifter's goals, competition pathway, time that can be given over to training and recovery, psychological and physical condition. For example, an athlete with a particular weakness may stay in Phase 2 for four weeks and Phase 3 for two weeks. On the other hand there may only be twelve weeks available to make gains between key competitions. Consequently, the phases should be divided according to aims and targets that have been discussed and set with all concerned.

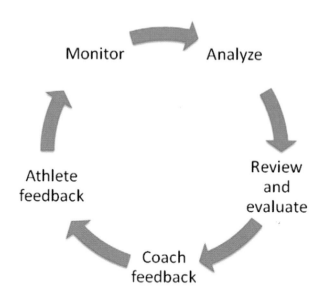

Critical factors to success.

Stages of Training

Stage 1: De-load phase

This stage can last anything from ten days to four weeks and generally far less weight is lifted. The block of training often consists of strength and conditioning and pre-hab work, encompassing a group of exercises which extend from physiotherapy. An example of this would be more specific pole work movements such as stretching the hip flexors, performing half squats (as opposed to full squats) for gluteus firing. These exercises are designed to strengthen the athlete's weak links and prevent injury. They are highly athlete-specific and are a product of both physiotherapist and coach consultations.

All training sessions in this phase will be devised and linked together to facilitate recovery from the previous heavy loading the body will have undertaken. The sessions are often a combination of light weight training, possibly with machines, and may introduce some low impact aerobic work such as a swimming session. When possible, a whole time slot usually reserved for heavy powerlifting training may be spent with a service provider instead, such as a nutritionist. The key is to introduce active rest and help the athlete mentally and physically re-charge and work on weaker underlying areas. Again, this is athlete-specific and is usually linked to finance; if the lifter is not in a position to access specific support for this phase it would be advisable to take a little time off after a heavy and/or challenging training cycle.

Such blocks of athlete-centred training are best prescribed via a conditioning coach in conjunction with a physiotherapist, while taking on board the powerlifting coach's assessment from the previous training cycle. Remember, weakness will be easily identifiable by working through the lifter's training diary.

An example of a week in the de-load phase

Prior to commencing each lifting session the athlete should complete 1000m on a rowing

Table 2   Example of a week in de-load phase

Day 1	Day 2	Day 3	Day 4	Day 5	Day 6	Day 7
Session 1 Aqua jogging – 20 minutes	**Session 1 Bench Press** 3 × 12 at 65–75% of Comp. bench	**REST DAY** **Session 1** Physiotherapy or massage	**Session 1 Narrow grip bench** (triceps) 3 × 12 at 60%	**Session 1 Back Squats** 3 × 12 at 60–65% (of Comp. Squat)	**Session 1 Power walking** 30 minutes	**Session 1 Pole work** 3 × 8 each leg
Session 2 Nutritionist	**Deep dumbbell press** 3 × 10		**Band triceps pull downs** 3 × 12	**Stiff leg deadlifts (light)** 3 × 10	**Session 2 Pole work –** full body stretching	**Light front squats** 3 × 10
	Dumbbell shoulder press sitting on Swiss ball 3 × 8		**Seated rows (light)** 3 × 10–12	**Lunges** 3 × 8	**Core – weighted Swiss ball crunches** 4 × 10	**Single leg press** 3 × 10 (each leg)
			Wide grip lat pull downs 3 × 12	**Seated calf raises** 3 × 10		**Bicep curls** 3 × 10
	Rotary cuffs with light band – front and side raises 3 × 10 each way		**Crunches** No weight 5 × 10	**Full body stretch**	**Standing oblique cable rotations** 4 × 10	
			Cross over crunches 3 × 8		**Cross over crunches** 3 × 8	
			Hanging leg raises 3 × 10		Or equivalent core session	

machine (or equivalent) and full body stretches. Post-session they should perform full body stretches.

Repeat and adjust progressively. As with any training programme, each week will be progressive where possible, usually by adding sets and reps. This stage should align with the lifter's competition schedule.

As the training progresses it will become evident that more components are added and that the number and intensity of the sets and reps to be performed increases at the same time. Therefore, it is imperative to note that whenever one element of activity is added, two elements of recovery are also added.

Stage 2

Review the athlete's conditioning and readiness to undertake a new training cycle and begin data analysis. Re-introduce the three to five main training sessions per week (if they have been cut down in the previous phase). Start to add intermediate levels of skill and increase the intensity of the resistance within the weight-bearing exercises, and increase the degree of difficulty of the technical aspects of the lift. This may mean breaking down the lifts into part lifts, for example performing squats to a Swiss ball or placing a board on the chest to alter and decrease the range of movement when bench pressing. To increase the ranges of movement of the deadlift, ask the lifter to stand on blocks whilst performing the exercise.

For the lifter described above, prescribe pole work sessions three times a week to simulate the bench press movement followed by practising the bench press arch position once a week whilst holding the loaded bar at 75 per cent in the start position for thirty seconds at a time – see the formula below:

Arch holds exercise
(number of sets × duration)
Week 1: 2 × 30 seconds
Week 2: 3 × 30 seconds
Week 3: 3 × 30 seconds

(From here on add time rather than sets using increments of 5–10 seconds according to how the lifter adapts.)

Week 4: 3 × 40 seconds

This continues to increase until the lifter is able to complete 3 × 60 seconds, at which point they would reduce the time to 40 seconds, add another set and increase the weight by 5 per cent, for example 4 × 40 seconds holding 80 per cent. The long-term aim would be to complete 5 × 60 seconds with 110 per cent of 1RM bench press.

For this particular lifter introduce quarter deadlifts standing on 8cm high blocks or a step. The object here is to extend the lifting range. To achieve this put the loaded bar on a platform or wooden block so that the lifter starts the 'pull' from just below the knee rather than from the floor. Film the top part of the deadlift, play it back to the athlete, coach them so they can see and understand when and why they shrug or stand up to full extension and the completion of the lift.

Apply the same principle to the squat in order to ascertain at which point the bar begins to travel down the torso during the lift. For the lifter in this case study this is at 85 per cent of the 1RM. In effect the range of movement is shorter and gradually increases to full range.

Continue to work on the surrounding muscle groups and part movements and slowly begin to increase the amount of loading at the weakest point that is being addressed.

Start training specific muscle groups and muscle combinations to improve body composition as well as continuing to improve the three lifts. Include legs, hamstrings, quads, calves, triceps, chest upper and lower, shoulders front, back and rotary cuffs, back upper and lower.

Powerlifters are known for not including biceps as a prime muscle. Nevertheless they do require a relative level of conditioning. Hence it is advisable to include them in stages 1–3. It is also important to include a comprehensive core programme.

An example of Week 1 in Stage 2
Prior to commencing each weights session complete 1000m on a rowing machine (or equivalent) and full body stretches. Post-session, perform full body stretches. Add full core session a minimum of twice a week.

Table 3 Week 1 Stage 2

Day 1	Day 2	Day 3	Day 4	Day 5	Day 6	Day 7
Session 1 Aqua jogging –20 minutes	**Session 1 Pole work –** simulating bench press movement	**REST DAY**	**Session 1 Pole work –** simulating bench press movement and overhead squat	**Session 1 Back Squats** 4 × 8 at 75% – 80%	**ACTIVE REST**	**Session 1 Pole work –** simulating bench press movement and overhead squat
Session 2 Pole work – simulating bench press movement	**Board press (bench)** 3 × 10 at approximately 70%	**Session 1** Physio or massage		**Leg press** 5 × 5 (heavy)	**Session 1 Power walking** 30 minutes	
Step ups with 5kg dumbbells in each hand 3 × 8 each leg	**Fast bench**** 3 grips: 3 × 10 wide 3 × 10 medium 3 × 10 narrow		**Narrow grip bench (triceps)** 3 × 10	**Stiff leg dead lifts** 3 × 10	**Session 2** Review session with coach	**Practise the arch** 2 × 3 –30 seconds
			Triceps extensions (with dumbbells) 3 × 12	**Seated calf raises** 3 × 10	**Session 3 Pole work –** full body stretching	**Quarter dead lifts** 3 × 8
Box squats* 3 × 8 at 65%	**Reverse files** 3 × 10			**Full body stretch**		
Bicep curls 3 × 10			**Triceps bench dips** 3 × 10–12			**Sumo deadlift** 3 × 8
	Wide grip lat pull downs 3 × 8		**Upright rows** 3 × 8			
Session 3 Nutritionist						**Prone rows** 3 × 8
	Rotary cuff With light band – front and side raises 3 × 10 each way		**Dumbbell shoulder press** sitting on Swiss ball 3 × 8			

Key to secondary exercises:

*Box squats: back squat to a bench that has been pre-set at just below parallel. Hold position on the bench without sitting (similar to a pause during a bench press), then return to standing.

**Fast bench: bring the bar down to the chest, then under control push the bar back up evenly through both arms to the start position as fast as possible (without pausing on the chest).

Stage 3

At this point, ascertaining the athlete's optimal recovery regime is key. Introduce recovery methods such as heat and ice and cryo-cuffs and, if possible, increase the use of massage. Perhaps by altering training times, try to fit in a power nap or rest period during the day (this could include sitting in the car with a relaxation tape in the lunch hour at work). Monitor the effects of going to bed early two nights per week. A simple way to measure any differences to training output would be to retire early the night before a heavy session or retire early the night after a heavy training session.

Review, reflect and analyze all the captured data from the previous two stages. If possible increase work on sports psychology, consolidate the nutrition plan and increase loading on secondary exercises (exercises targeting the muscle groups that support the three lifts).

Vary the secondary exercises to alleviate boredom. Increase the level of technical conditioning (including skill). This will encompass work with the skeletal frame and muscle groups working in unison to hold the starting position of the lifts. Employ basic biomechanics and, where possible, utilize computer software to track the pathway of the bar during the three lifts. Top lifters will add chains and bands to the loaded bar to create different dimensions and types of resistance to their training. Aim for visible improvement of technique and lifting aptitude.

If possible add in an extra powerlifting training day into a seven or ten day training rotation week.

Stage 4
Week 1: Working to 80 per cent of previous best lift

Note at this stage the primary goal is to prepare the athlete to compete. As such, the focus now becomes the execution of the three lifts whilst progressively increasing the weights and reducing the repetitions.

Any secondary exercises vary by lifter and are selected in line the individual's strengths and recovery status. Hence the secondary exercises have been selected specially for the athlete introduced above.

If the proposed starting weight is too heavy build in a lighter set of ascending warm-up sets and exercises. For example, on the deadlift 2 × 10 at 30kg, 1 × 5 at 50kg, then follow the programme below. As this programme is a real life example, at times the weight denominations increase by increments of 1kg, for example 35kg to 36kg. This is achieved by using 500g discs to make up the 1kg denomination. If these are not available, adjust accordingly, for example go up with less weight and add one more set.

Fine-tune mental skills and work towards narrowing the focus on the three lifts, the weight to be lifted and the style in which the lifts are to be achieved during competition

Table 4   Week 1 Stage 4

Day 1	Day 2	Day 3	Day 4	Day 5	Day 6	Day 7
Session 1 Powerlifting (PL) back squat	**Session 1 Pole work**	**REST DAY**	**Session 1**	**ACTIVE REST**	**Session 1** Nutritionist/ establish body weight	**REST DAY**
1 × 8 – 50kg		**Session 1**	**Traditional deadlift**			**Make sure training and food diaries are up to date**
1 × 4 – 65kg	**Competition style bench press**	Massage or physio	1 × 6 – 60kg	**Session 1** Abdominal exercises		
1 × 2 – 80kg	2 × 10 – 20kg		1 × 3 – 80 kg		**Session 2 Box Squats**	
6 × 3 – 95kg	1 × 6 – 35kg	**Session 2** Sports psychologist	1 × 1 – 95kg		(wide stance) 3 × 10 at 65% of PB of box squat	
	1 × 5 – 45kg		1 × 1 – 105kg	Stretching and pole work		
Leg press	5 × 5 – 60kg		6 × 3 – 115kg			
3 × 10 (moderate weight –aim for full range of movement)	**Rack press*** 5 × 6 – 45kg (flat back no arch)		**Sumo dead lift** 3 × 8 – 80kg	**Session 2** Walking on a treadmill or equivalent	**Leg extensions** 3 × 8	
Step ups (with a Powerlifting bar loaded to 30kg) 3 × 10 each leg	**Incline dumbbell press** 3 × 8 – (10kg in each hand)		**Wide grip pull downs** 3 × 10		**Stiff leg deadlift** 3 × 10 – 25kg	
Upright rows 3 × 10 – 35kg	**Prone rows** 5 × 6 – 30 kg				**Narrow grip bench**** with band on the bar 3 × 8 – 35kg	
Front and side lateral raises 5kg in each hand 3 × 8 each way	**Back stretches** off Swiss ball 3 × 8 (no weight)				**Triceps extensions with bar** 3 × 10 – 20kg	
Session 2 Review with coach					**Triceps machine pushdowns** 3 × 10	

Key to secondary exercises:

***Rack press:** The powerlifting bar is placed at the lifter's sticking point on a rack across the chest, and the lifter then bench presses from this starting point.

****Narrow grip bench with band looped to the bar:** This is accomplished by looping the band a number of times round the end of the bar, done to add extra resistance; the tighter the band, the greater the resistance.

The lifter should note their body weight, both first thing in the morning and in the evening. Calculate what is required either to decrease or increase weight and the type and amounts of supplements required for the athlete to complete the training programme and recover sufficiently to go about their daily life between training sessions. At this point the lifter in this case study will now be talking to a nutritionist on a weekly basis.

Table 5   Week 2 Stage 4

Day 1	Day 2	Day 3	Day 4	Day 5	Day 6	Day 7
Session 1 PL squat 1 × 8 – 50kg 1 × 4 – 65kg 1 × 2 – 80kg 6 × 4 – 95kg	**Session 1 Comp. bench press** 2 × 10 – 20kg 1 × 6 – 30kg 1 × 5 – 42.5kg 1 × 3 – 52.5kg 1 × 2 – 57.5kg 5 × 5 – 62.5kg	**REST DAY** **Session 1** Massage or physio **Session 2** Sports psychologist	**Session 1 Traditional deadlift** 1 × 6 – 60kg 1 × 2 –80kg 1 × 1 – 95kg 1 × 2 – 105kg 6 × 4 – 115kg	**ACTIVE REST** **Session 1** Abdominal exercises Stretching and pole work	**Session 1 Box Squats** *(wide stance)* 3 × 10 *at 70% of PB of box squat*	**REST DAY** **Make sure training and food diaries are up to date**
Leg press 3 × 10	**Rack press** 5 × 5 – 47kg		**Sumo deadlift** 3 × 8 –85kg	**Session 2** Walking on a treadmill or equivalent. Increase time by 2 minutes	**Leg extensions** 4 × 8	
Step ups *(with a Powerlifting bar loaded to 30kg)* 3 × 10 each leg	**Incline dumbbell press** 3 × 8 – 10kg in each hand		**Wide grip pull downs** 3 × 10		**Stiff leg deadlift** 3 × 10 – 27kg	
Upright rows 4 × 10 – 35kg	**Prone rows** 5 × 5 – 32kg				**Narrow grip bench** *with band on the bar* 3 × 8 – 35kg	
Front and side lateral raises –5 kg in each hand 3 × 8 each way	**Back stretches** *off Swiss ball* 3 × 8 *(no weight)*				**Triceps extensions with bar** 4 × 10	
Session 2 Review with coach					**Triceps machine push downs** 3 × 10	

Be sure to book into the competition, fill out all documentation and send off the entry fee.

Table 6   Week 3 Stage 4

Day 1	Day 2	Day 3	Day 4	Day 5	Day 6	Day 7
Session 1 PL squat 1 × 8 – 50kg 1 × 4 – 65kg 1 × 2 – 80kg 6 × 5 – 95kg	**Session 1 Comp. bench press** 2 × 10 – 20kg 1 × 6 – 30kg 1 × 5 – 42.5kg 1 × 3 – 52.5kg 1 × 2 – 60kg 4 × 4 – 65kg	**REST DAY** **Session 1** Massage or physio **Session 2** Sports psychologist	**Session 1** Review previous footage of lifts **Session 2 Deadlift** 1 × 6 – 60kg 1 × 2 – 80kg 1 × 1 – 95kg 1 × 1 – 105kg 6 × 5 – 110kg	**ACTIVE REST** **Session 1** Stretching and pole work **Session 2** Performance lifestyle advisor	**Session 1 Box Squats** *(medium stance)* 3 × 8 *at 72% of PB of box squat*	**REST DAY** **Make sure training and food diaries are up to date**
Step ups *(with a PL bar 32kg)* 3 × 8 each leg	**Rack press** 5 × 4 – 50kg		**Traditional deadlift (on blocks)** 3 × 8 –80kg	**Session 3** Walking on a treadmill or equivalent.	**Leg extensions** 4 × 6 **Stiff leg deadlift** 3 × 8 – 30kg	**Confirm body weight** **Stock up on any supplements that may be required**
Upright rows 5 × 8 – 35kg **Front and side lateral raises** –5kg in each hand 3 × 8 each way	**Decline dumbbell press** 3 × 8 – 8kg in each hand **Prone rows** 4 × 4 – 35kg		**Wide grip pull downs** 3 × 10		**Narrow grip bench** *with band on the bar** add an extra loop* 3 × 6 – 36kg	
Session 2 Review with coach	**Back stretches** *off Swiss ball* 3 × 8 *(no weight)*				**Triceps extensions with bar only** 4 × 10 **Triceps machine push downs** 4 × 10	

Table 7   Week 4 Stage 4

Day 1	Day 2	Day 3	Day 4	Day 5	Day 6	Day 7
Session 1 Abdominal exercises stretching and pole work	**Session 1 Comp. bench press** 2 × 10 – 20kg 1 × 6 – 32kg 1 × 4 – 40kg 1 × 3 – 50kg 1 × 2 – 57.5kg 1 × 2 – 62.5kg 4 × 4 – 67.5kg	**REST DAY** **Session 1** Massage or physio	**Session 1 Deadlift** 1 × 6 – 60kg 1 × 2 – 80kg 1 × 1 – 95kg 1 × 1 – 105kg 6 × 6 – 115kg	**ACTIVE REST** **Session 1** Aqua jogging	**Session 1 Box Squats** *(medium stance)* 3 × 8 *at 75% of PB of box squat*	**REST DAY** **Make sure training and food diaries are up to date**
PL squat 1 × 8 – 50kg 1 × 4 – 65kg 1 × 2 – 80kg 6 × 6 – 95kg	**Slow wide grip bench** *(3 second pause)* 3 × 8 – 45kg	**Session 2** Filming body alignment whilst doing pole work	**Traditional deadlift (on blocks)** 3 × 8 – 85kg	**Session 2** Abdominalls, Stretching and pole work	**Leg extensions** 5 × 6	**Confirm body weight**
Step ups *(with a PL bar 32kg)* 4 × 8 each leg	**Decline dumbbell press** 4 × 8 – 8kg *in each hand*	**Session 3** Sports psychologist	**Wide grip pull downs** 4 × 10	**Session 3** Review footage from Day 3	**Stiff leg deadlift** 3 × 8 – 32kg **Narrow grip bench** *with band on the bar** 5 × 6 – 36kg	**Confirm competition entry and check that all kit is both functional and will pass a kit check**
Upright rows 5 × 8 – 35kg	**Prone rows** 4 × 4 – 35kg				**Triceps extensions with bar only** 4 × 10	
Front and side lateral raises –5kg *in each hand* 3 × 10 each way	**Back stretches** *off Swiss ball* 4 × 8 *(no weight)*				**Triceps machine push downs** 5 × 8 *(increase weight)*	
Session 3 Review with coach						

Be clear about the competition logistics, for example weigh-in time and mode, and timing of transport for travelling to the venue.

Table 8   Week 5 Stage 4

Day 1	Day 2	Day 3	Day 4	Day 5	Day 6	Day 7
Session 1 Abdominal exercises, stretching and pole work	**Session 1 Comp. Bench:** 2 × 10 – 20kg 1 × 6 – 32kg 1 × 4 – 40kg 1 × 3 – 50kg 1 × 2 – 57.5kg 1 × 2 – 62.6kg 4 × 4 – 67.5kg	**REST DAY** **Session 1** Physio or massage	**Session 1 Deadlift** 1 × 6 – 70kg 1 × 2 – 90kg 1 × 2 – 105kg 4 × 4 – 117.5kg 1 × 4 – 122.5kg 1 × 4 – 130kg	**ACTIVE REST** **Session 1** Aqua jogging	**Session 1 Box Squats** (medium stance) 3 × 8 (at 80% of PB of Box Squat)	**REST DAY** **Make sure training and food diaries are up to date**
PL squat 1 × 8 – 40 kg 1 × 4 – 55kg 1 × 2 – 70kg 1 × 1 – 85kg 4 × 4 – 100kg	**Slow wide grip bench** (3 second pause) 4 × 8 – 45kg	**Session 2** Sports psychologist	**Traditional deadlift on blocks** 4 × 8 –85kg	**Session 2** Abdominals, stretching and pole work	**Leg extensions** 5 × 6	**Confirm body weght**
Step ups (with a Powerlifting bar loaded to 35kg) 5 × 6 each leg	**Decline dumbell press** 4 × 8 –8kg	**Session 3** Nutritionist	**Wide grip lat pull downs** 5 × 8 (keep form)	**Session 3** Review training diary	**Stiff leg Deadlift** 4 × 8 – 32kg	**Confirm competition entry and check that all kit is both functional and will pass a kit check**
Upright rows 5 × 5 – 37.5kg	**Prone rows** 4 × 4 –37kg				**Narrow grip bench** (with band on the bar) 5 × 5 – 40kg	
Front and side lateral raises – 5 kg in each hand 3 × 10 each way	**Back extensions** (off Swiss ball) 3 × 8 (with 5kg disc)				**Triceps extensions with bar** 4 × 10 – 20kg	
Review with coach					**Triceps machine push downs** 5 × 8 (as last week)	

Table 9   Week 6 Stage 4

Day 1	Day 2	Day 3	Day 4	Day 5	Day 6	Day 7
Session 1 Abdominal exercises, stretching and pole work	**Session 2 Comp. Bench:** 2 × 10 – 20kg 1 × 6 – 32kg 1 × 4 – 40kg 1 × 3 – 50kg 1 × 2 – 57.5kg	**REST DAY** **Session 1** Physio or massage	**Session 1 Deadlift** 1 × 6 – 60kg 1 × 2 – 80kg 1 × 2 – 95kg 1 × 2 – 105kg 1 × 1 – 115kg 3 × 3 – 130kg	**ACTIVE REST** **Session 1** Aqua jogging	**Session 1 Box Squats** (medium stance) 4 × 8 (at 80% of PB of Box Squat)	**REST DAY** **Make sure training and food diaries are up to date**
PL squat 1 × 8 – 40 kg 1 × 4 – 60g 1 × 2 – 75kg 1 × 1 – 90kg 3 × 3 – 105kg	1 × 2 – 62.5kg 1 × 2 – 67.5kg 2 × 2 – 72.5kg	**Session 2** Sports psychologist	1 × 3 – 140kg 1 × 3 – 145kg	**Session 2** Abdominals, stretching and pole work	**Stiff leg Deadlift** 4 × 8 – 32kg	**Confirm body weght**
Step ups (with a Powerlifting bar loaded to 35kg) 5 × 6 each leg	**Deep dumbell press** 3 × 8 –10kg in each hand	**Session 3** Nutritionist	**Traditional deadlift on blocks** 4 × 8 –90kg **Wide grip lat pull downs** 5 × 8 (keep form)	**Session 3** Review training diary	**Narrow grip bench** (with band on the bar) 5 × 5 – 41kg	**Confirm competition entry and check that all kit is both functional and will pass a kit check**
Leg curls 3 × 10	**Back extensions** (off Swiss ball) 3 × 8 (with 5kg disc)				**Triceps extensions with bar only** 5 × 8	
Rotary cuff stretches with light resistance band 3 × 8					**Triceps machine push downs** 5 × 8 (as last week)	
Review with coach						

The athlete should let the coach and nutritionist know if they are struggling with body weight. They can advise and adjust calorie intake, recovery and training to bring the process back in line. Teamwork helps here.

Table 10 Week 7 Stage 4

Day 1	Day 2	Day 3	Day 4	Day 5	Day 6	Day 7
Session 1 Formal Squat 1 × 8 – 45kg 1 × 4 – 60kg 1 × 2 – 70kg 1 × 2 – 80kg 1 × 1 – 95kg 2 × 2 – 112.5kg	**Session 1 Comp. Bench** 2 × 10 – 20kg 1 × 6 – 32kg 1 × 4 – 40kg 1 × 3 – 50kg 1 × 2 – 57.5kg 1 × 1 – 65kg 1 × 1 – 70kg 2 × 1 – 72.5kg	**REST DAY** **Session 1** Physio or massage	**Session 1 Deadlift** 1 × 6 – 70kg 1 × 2 – 85kg 1 × 2 – 100kg 1 × 1 – 120kg 2 × 2 – 130kg 1 × 2 – 140kg 1 × 2 – 150kg	**FULL REST DAY** Practise mental skills training	**Session 1 Box Squats** (medium stance) 4 × 6 (at 85% of PB of Box Squat)	**Session 1** Massage
Lunges 3 × 10		**Session 2** Sports psychologist	**'A' bar Lat pull downs** 3 × 8		**Stiff leg Deadlift** 4 × 4 – 40kg	**Session 2** Practise mental skills training
Review with coach Be sure of logistical arrangements for competition	**Deep dumbell press** 3 × 8 –10kg (each hand)	**Session 3** Nutritionist **Session 4** Session with coach to discuss competition strategy	**Single arm dumbbell rows** 3 × 8 (each arm)		**Narrow grip bench** (with band on the bar) 5 × 6 – 41kg	**Session 3** Review food diary with nutritionist **Session 4** Check all personal equipment and competition logistics
Be sure of body weight	**Incline press with bar** 3 × 10 at 35kg				**Triceps extensions with bar only** 5 × 8	
					Triceps machine push downs 5 × 8 (as last week)	

Table 11 Week 8 Stage 4

Day 1	Day 2	Day 3	Day 4	Day 5	Day 6	Day 7
Session 1 Formal Squat Up to 2 × 1 – 110g	**REST DAY Session 1** Sports psychologist	**REST DAY** **Session 1 Com. Bench press** 3 × 6 – 45kg	**ACTIVE REST Full body stretching** **No cardio unless required for body weight**	**REST DAY** **Session 1** Mental skills rehearsal for competition	**Competition day** *Opening lifts – always subject to change on the day*	**REST DAY** for athlete Coach to review competition
Lat pull downs 3 × 10 *(light)*		**Dumbbell press** 3 × 8 – with resistance band			**Squat:** Opening attempt – 110kg	
Seated rows 3 × 10 *(light)*		**Leg press** 3 × 8 at 60%			**Bench Press:** Opening attempt – 67.5kg	
					Deadlift: Opening attempt – 147.5kg	

CHAPTER 6

TRAINING DIARIES

To monitor progression and see how the training programme is working, the coach is likely to introduce a training diary. Training diaries have become popular and invaluable tools for athletes at all levels. They range from hard copy calendar-style diaries to the state-of-the art, sport-specific electronic diaries used by Olympians, Paralympians and professional sports people.

The purpose of a training diary is to collect and record data on the training attempted and completed and to capture the daily aspects of the athlete's training regime. One of its most practical uses is to act as a 'mirror' since it often highlights a discrepancy between what the athlete thinks they have accomplished (effort) and what they have actually achieved (output) and enables them to make beneficial adjustments to their training activity.

Benefits of a Training Diary

* Establishes baseline data which can be used by all involved (athlete, coach, parent, service providers), with informed consent.
* Enables realistic, obtainable goals to be set, with corresponding timelines.
* Enables lifters and coaches to work with facts, not guesswork.
* Enables comparisons and analyses to be carried out.
* Reveals patterns in training dips and Personal Best performances.
* Identifies highs and lows in mood, as well as lifestyle changes.

* Makes it easier to distinguish patterns of events that contribute to competition results.
* Helps an athlete to establish how far they have progressed from their baseline and how near they are to achieving their goals.
* Helps to narrow and re-align the training focus.
* Enables the athlete to better understand where powerlifting fits into their life and what route they want to follow in the sport.
* Identifies how the athlete may respond to different stimuli.
* Enables all components of performance to be tracked and priorities realigned to help the athlete achieve the best possible outcomes.
* Helps build a portfolio of evidence that can be used to persuade potential sponsors or GB selection panels that the athlete is capable of delivering to their targets.

As well as their invaluable role in helping the athlete and all who work with them, powerlifting training diaries are also beneficial for the sport in the long run, as the rich data captured will help the sport to devise a template for creating a championship pathway.

Diary Formats

Diary formats vary considerably, and the decision on which one to use is a matter of personal choice. If an athlete opts for a smart phone app they would be well advised to save some of their historical training data on to their PC for backup purposes. Their data is valuable and if it is lost from a mobile device, it is gone for good. It is also worthwhile transferring any numerical data into a database or spreadsheet so that data analysis can be performed more easily. At the same time, it is recommended that athletes use word processing or spreadsheet software for the written elements of their diary as this will enable them to carry out more complex analysis and create graphical outputs, for instance by turning data into graphs and performance curves.

If handwriting in a hard copy diary seems like a chore and working with electronic applications is either not possible or simply tiresome, the athlete should find or create a method or template that suits them. For example, they could use a simple rating chart in which they score their training sessions by applying different coloured faces with varying expressions and use numbers to rate each segment of the session.

A training diary is the athlete's personal tool. Its purpose is to benefit them and their performance. They should use the format that best suits them and their learning style, and record their data in a way that is meaningful to them and useful for the coach. If happy and sad faces work, then that is the correct format.

Measuring scales
Here are some suggested measuring scales that can be used singly or in combination to accommodate all learning styles.

Letters and numbers
Session A = 5 (excellent)
Session B = 4 (good)
Session C = 3 (poor)

An example of a personal handwritten training diary showing details of a training session (May 11, 2011).

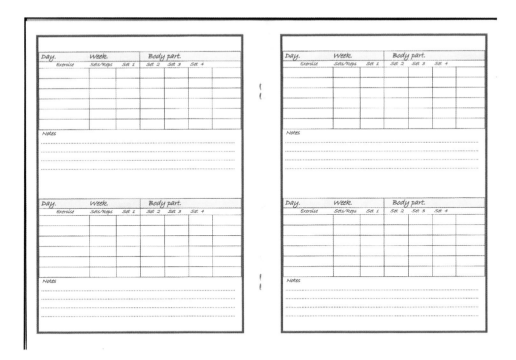

ABOVE: An example of a templated training diary.

BELOW: An example from the BluePrint for Success© electronic athlete/coach diary.

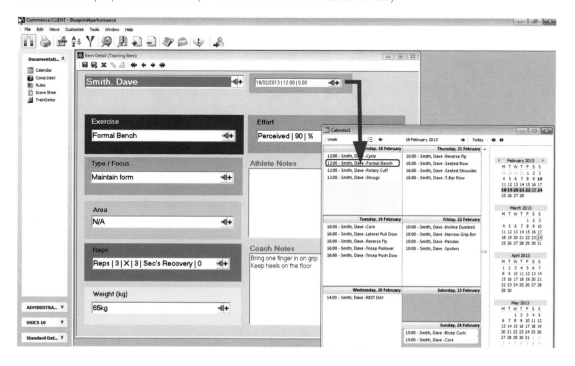

Pictorial
Green happy face (= excellent)
Amber neutral face (= good)
Red sad face (= poor)

Linear

	Mood scale	
High		Low
	8-7	
10	5	0

Mood scale.

I choose to use a mood scale, as mood has been shown to affect lifters' quality of training. In my opinion powerlifters are often best positioned between seven and eight on the scale (that is, 'good') to allow them to train well. I have observed that if the athletes are demonstrating over-euphoric behaviour they may find it difficult to apply the technical elements of their training that have not yet become second nature, and in this mood state lifting can appear erratic. Conversely if a lifter feels too low, apathy can set in which can lead to low self-esteem, all of which can affect behaviour and attitude towards a training session or competition.

Capturing Data

When an athlete introduces a training diary into their life it is far better to collect less data accurately than end up with big gaps or made-up entries. The first thing to capture is what happens in each training session, noting that every session requires a rationale and should be a building block towards the overall performance outcome. At the very least the daily entry of any training diary should record in full the warm-up, the weights lifted, the sets and reps attempted and those completed. It should also record the duration of the session and if the training was completed as prescribed and, if not, how it differed.

Other data for a daily diary
- Body weight (it is best for the athlete to weigh on the same scales, on the same day and at the same time of day each week).
- Levels of tiredness pre- and post-session.
- Sleep rated by quality and quantity.
- Hydration levels (measured by using a urine chart).
- Any restrictive movement noted in the joints or niggles that may be the prelude to injury.
- Muscle soreness or tightness.
- The athlete's thoughts on whether they felt able to lift more weight than prescribed.
- Mood
- Female athletes to record menstrual cycle.

Regular Review of Diary Entries

It is a good idea for the athlete to read through their diary on a regular basis and reflect on the entries. They should think about what they entered and what they felt at the time. Did they forget to mention something that might be important? For example, perhaps they tried a different type of recovery drink or found themselves stuck in traffic for an hour longer than normal when travelling to the gym. How did this make them feel? Both coach and athlete should consider any anomalies. For example, if the athlete felt unusually tired during a particular session could this have been due to the fact that they took on more home chores two days previously? If they recorded an excellent session could this have been due to the fact that they enjoyed three good nights' sleep in a row? By recording their training activities and reviewing them in the context of their daily life, both the coach and the athlete can build up a valuable picture of some of the elements that may affect the athlete's lifting performance.

At the end of each block of training it is a good idea to review and analyze the training programme. Consider if there has been some adaptation – a measurable and positive physical or mental change. This is not always as obvious as managing to lift more weight on the bar when executing one of the three lifts as it will depend on what component the athlete has been focusing on. For instance, they may want to achieve a 10 per cent increase on the weight to be lifted before the knees travel too far towards the toes during the descent of the squat. This would be measured at the onset of the training block and tracked during specific training sessions.

Injury History

No athlete can afford to be injured, and a training diary can aid early detection of weak points and stressors. Logging as much information as possible about all injuries incurred will assist in any medical handover, both post-injury and during the transition from the re-hab phase to the pre-hab phase. It will also help to ensure the continuity of care provided by medical staff and coaches.

Capturing injury data
The athlete should:

- Note down the date and location of the incident.
- Provide a brief explanation of how it happened.
- Record the actual diagnosis of the injury and the treatment prescribed and/or undertaken.
- Record any medication taken, including exact dose times (see Chapter 10).
- List all drugs taken, where and when.

The following sequence demonstrates how the athlete's injury data may be captured via electronic athlete/coach diary for use by the appointed service providers (in this example the physiotherapist).

Competition Record and History

However the athlete chooses to capture their

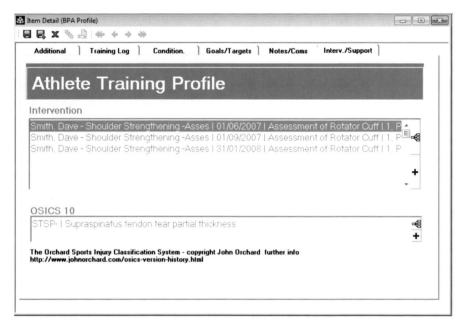

An example from the BluePrint for Success© electronic athlete/ coach diary, showing that the athlete has a partial tear in their supraspinatus tendon; a classification of that injury; and three appointments the athlete has had with the physio.

Intervention item showing details of one of the appointments and the assessment items carried out by the physio. BluePrint for Success©

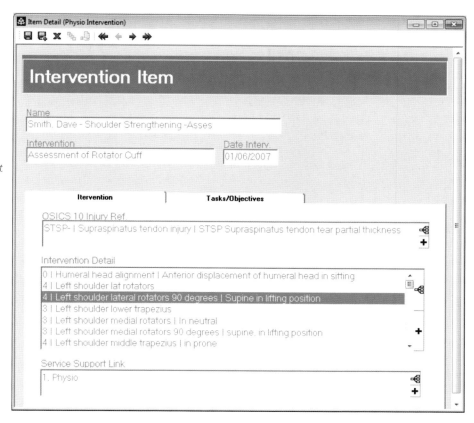

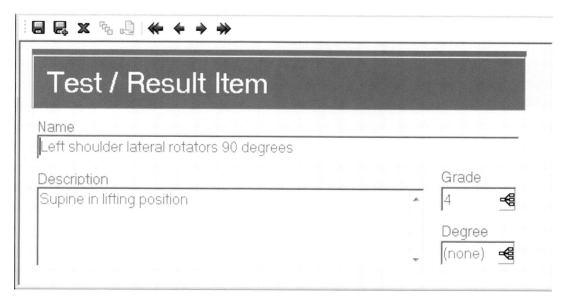

Test/result item showing one of the test elements that the physio has carried out. BluePrint for Success©

data it is a good idea to keep a record of all the competitions they have entered with the corresponding results. Below is an example of a template that could be filled in post-competition.

- The location of the competition (distance to be travelled by the athlete).
- Outcome goals.
- Body weight.
- Number of lights per lift given.
- Number of successful lifts.
- Achievement of outcome goals.
- What went well and what could have been done better?

Completing the diary with a descriptive narrative that is meaningful to the athlete, that charts their targets and competition history as well as their behaviours and reactions to particular situations, will build a picture of their critical success factors. By cross-referencing this with all the other dimensions they have been recording along the way (including their lifestyle and support network), the athlete will be in a position to create a progressive, effective and manageable plan for their next training cycle.

Showing the Broad Picture

By maintaining a training diary the athlete is building a history of all the training prescribed and completed and creating a blueprint for their growth and success as a lifter. The diary will reveal a wide range of valuable information including insights into personal traits, both good and bad. Sleep patterns will emerge; lifestyle choices to be made will become apparent.

The diary could help the athlete determine if they are going through the motions when training or if they have, in fact, reached a 'glass ceiling' and need to make informed choices in order to move forward in one direction or another. Armed with all this information the athlete will be able to identify the actions they need to take to proceed along their chosen pathway and to anticipate and manage some of the inevitable challenges that will arise. For example the data collected over a period of time may indicate that, to be competitive at the next tier above, the athlete needs to add an extra training session per week, the focus of which should be strength and conditioning as opposed to simply repeating what they

---

EXCERPTS FROM LIFTERS' TRAINING DIARIES

'I know what I have to do and will do it.'

'I will come back stronger.'

'My legs felt like jelly before the first squat, never really got it together until the deadlifts. Did get a PB on last lift. Need to be able to pull all the lifts together on the day.'

'Feels like forever when waiting for the competition to begin.'

'Feeling quiet today, like I can't remember home any more…' (athlete had been away for ten days attending a world championships).

'I can't take much more of the same food choices every day – even though the food is of a good quality.'
'Feel like I have too much energy today – need to train.'

'Not feeling too good today, nothing seemed to go right.'

'Had a brilliant session today.'

An example of a handwritten training diary showing the athlete's interpretation of their competition result (June 4, 2011). Note that for the three red lights at 80kg (fail) the lifter felt there was nothing wrong with their performance!

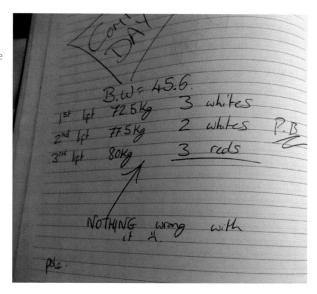

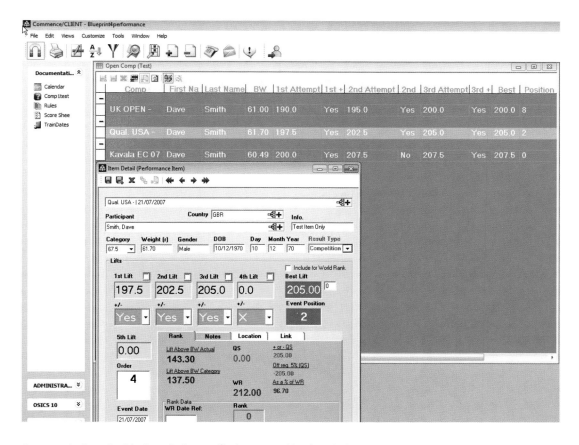

An example from the BluePrint for Success© electronic athlete/coach diary showing competition result.

are already doing i.e. they should add another element to their training.

Additionally, the athlete may identify a need for specific physiotherapy advice and some treatment sessions to help with flexibility. After thinking it through, the athlete could decide that this would place too much personal and financial strain on their family life under their current circumstances. Therefore, they may decide to place the family unit as their main priority and consider various options for obtaining physio service, for example by contacting their local practitioners who may be willing to offer some form of sponsorship.

Next, they may decide to shift the focus of two of their main powerlifting sessions to the technical aspects of lifting, keeping the rest the same. In this way they are able to continue to steadily improve in the areas of their choice while enjoying the sport and maintaining a lifestyle balance.

Another lifter faced with the same scenario may have a completely different lifestyle and commitments and may opt to take up the extra support and training session. Either way, collecting data via a training diary enables a lifter to become the best they can be by making informed choices and using the resources they have available to them at any point along their sporting journey.

Professional Training Diaries

Keeping a training log is an inherent part of the powerlifting culture, whether the data is captured in simple hard copy format or via a computer application. Any information gathered is for the use of the owner and whomever they choose to share it with.

While unfunded athletes may record their training information using any format they choose, such as making handwritten notes in a book, a funded athlete must log their data online in accordance with the requirements of their programme or professional body. This is for the sole purpose of aiding the athlete's performance, and the data will be shared across a whole team of coaches, service providers and medical teams, all of whom will have been vetted and will be required to comply with current data protection policy. In this way all the relevant parties can share their plans and expertise to identify and prioritize interventions, work efficiently as a team to deliver them and improve their athletes' overall sporting performance. Funded athletes will have these requirements fully explained to them and will need to sign a contract agreeing to data sharing.

One of the advantages of a professional funded system is that the coaches can upload the training programmes to a central system for their individual athletes to access. Other service providers who are supporting the athlete can also access the information and analyze the training. Meanwhile the athlete can pick up their training almost anywhere in the world at any time and receive up-to-the-minute changes and feedback. If they experience any difficulties or problems they can easily enter these into the system, alerting their support team, who will intervene accordingly. This can often help to prevent a minor incident becoming a major inhibitor to performance at a later date.

Linked to the training diary is a whole host of interactive web-based services such as notice boards and topical forums where athletes share tips and post ideas that have worked for them, for example a recipe for a milkshake they enjoyed which fitted within their nutritional regime. There are also international ranking lists, competition calendars and information on where to purchase equipment, together with state-of-the-art articles and journals, posted by coaches and service providers, and links to useful websites such as UK Sport and governing bodies.

Each sport has its own slant on the type of data to be recorded by its athletes and the channel/s for doing so. Since sport is constantly seeking ways to be leading edge, the approach to data capture is always evolving – today the emphasis may be on biomechanical analysis, tomorrow on chemical analysis. Whatever data is required, in whatever format, it all contributes to the delivery of a person-centred system that suits the athlete's learning style and supports the coach and service providers in helping the athlete achieve their goals.

The content of a full-time (funded) athlete's diary and the purpose to which the data is likely to be used will differ from a part-time (non-funded) athlete's due to the breadth and depth of data that must be captured by the former in order to create a complete picture of their progress. However, this does not mean that a part-time athlete will be any less committed to recording rich data that they can use to create a blueprint for their success.

Filling in the diary will take a little time to begin with. However, once it is part of the athlete's daily routine it will become easier and quicker to complete and may only take as little as five minutes per day. The review and analysis process will take a little longer, and it is suggested that the athlete sets aside half an hour a week to review the diary and perhaps one hour a month to extrapolate the main points and measure results against pre-set targets. The investment of time is extremely worthwhile as, by keeping a diary, the athlete is creating a personal manual for their sporting development.

PART 3

COMPETITION

CHAPTER 7

THE PROS AND CONS OF

COMPETING

The move from participation to competition in any sport has its advantages and disadvantages. All of these should be carefully considered when an athlete is deciding whether or not to compete. There is no right or wrong answer and the decision must be driven by what best suits the individual at a particular time in their life.

Reasons to Compete

Some lifters have a strong urge to pit their raw strength, acquired skill and mental toughness against their peers. For others it is a combination of reasons, for example the desire to improve their confidence or work through a plan to obtain an end goal.

It requires a great deal of hard work and commitment to become fit and able to compete, be it for a community level competition or a national championship. There is always a start point and an end point, the latter usually having a target attached to it. For some lifters the driving force is external, for example to lift as much weight as possible and thereby win the competition, which overrides any other factor. For others the driver could be internal, for example to build confidence.

Regardless, to lift well there has to be an equal measure of physical and mental application. Expressed as a formula, it would look something like this:

$$\text{(physical strength)} + \text{(body composition)} + \text{(cognitive application)} = \text{powerlifting}$$

Whether a lifter only competes once or enjoys a long, competitive career, entering a competition brings a sense of personal achievement, irrespective of the results. If the competition goes well and a total is gained, the lifter has a benchmark of the weights they have successfully lifted. On the other hand, if a total is not achieved but the lifter prepares properly and attempts the lifts in competition, they gain the respect of others for having the courage to compete. Gyms are full of individuals who trained for years and wished they had competed yet never actually did so.

The person who commits to and enters a competition will learn many valuable lessons. For example, they may discover that they do not enjoy competing but the experience shows them that they would prefer to train at this level and become a training partner for a competitive lifter. This way they can benefit from following progressive training plans without having to compete in public at the end of their training cycle.

Many lifters enjoy the escapism that comes from following a training programme and applying correct form in the gym. While focusing on this, there is no time to worry about life stresses such as paying the bills. Others enjoy the adrenalin rush that comes from competing, which is the main reason they compete. Many more enjoy the heightened sense of awareness that comes from competing in a safe, conducive and productive environment.

For an aspiring coach the process of preparing for and completing a powerlifting competition can be invaluable. Not only do they learn how to turn theoretical knowledge into practical application, they can use their personal experience of competing to support the lifters they will eventually coach.

Competing gives family and friends a chance to share in the passion by supporting the lifter at competitions. It also increases the lifter's social circle by including others who share the same passion, while opening up opportunities to network and share skills and ideas. For example, other lifters are usually happy to discuss their experience of using different types of personal equipment such as lifting suits, belts and knee wraps. Competitions are also a great place to try on and purchase equipment.

In addition, competitions provide a valuable opportunity to observe how experienced lifters maintain consistency of focus and good lifting technique, and learn how they manage nerves and adrenalin when gaining and failing lifts, and to consider how this affects their performance over the course of the event. Attending competitions as a spectator also provides valuable

insights into what referees are looking for during a lift, and it may be possible to speak to them during the breaks to ask for their perspective on a particular lifting style.

Whatever the level of competition, the sense of achievement will be the same. Having said that, each competition creates a unique experience. For example, in one competition a lifter may be aiming for a Personal Best while in another they may be trying out a different body weight class. Whatever the circumstances, the lifter is always pitting their physical strength against the bar and their technical execution of the lifts against the referee's opinion.

By competing, athletes develop their self-awareness and learn how to deliver against measurable pre-set goals. Competitions enable them to track their progress after all the hard work done in the gym, and even if this shows occasional stagnation they will have the chance to unpick why this is and move forward. Competing is a clear demonstration of strength of character, physical adaptation and mental and emotional aptitude, all of which are valuable transferable skills.

Remember no competition experience is wasted; many, many people train for years and never actually compete. Often, it is not the things you do that you regret but the things you don't do. So lift with your technique and let your passion drive you through the competition.

Disadvantages of Competing

To compete and be fully prepared to put in a credible performance requires full commitment. Training is time-consuming and lifters often feel very fatigued after a hard session in the gym. This, coupled with the need to rest and manage food intake, can impact negatively on social and family life.

These demands will be compounded by the financial implications of competing. Basic personal equipment must be purchased and there are gym fees and travel costs to be considered. It may also be necessary to buy better quality food and food supplements, all of which will add to the weekly budget.

If a lifter is selected for an international competition, but is unable able to secure funding or sponsorship, they often have to bear most of their travel costs themselves. Self-funding has long been a topic of debate within powerlifting because an athlete's ability to compete at the highest level may be, to a large extent, down to finance. There have been occasions when top-class lifters have been unable to compete due to lack of funds. Nevertheless, it should be remembered that it is still the best performer on the day who wins the competition and, as long as their lifts are ratified by the referees, there can be no argument that the competition is fair. As the popular saying goes: 'You have to be in it to win it'.

Competing requires many sacrifices. For instance, a sporting career can take up all annual leave from work because of the requirement to travel to training camps and competitions at home and abroad. If all this effort does not yield satisfying results the lifter may lose confidence and motivation and turn away from training altogether, which could have a negative impact on both health and fitness.

One of the problems that emerges with wanting to win at all costs is the temptation to take banned substances, which may increase the more successful a lifter becomes. This is an issue across all sports, and accordingly powerlifting is very well regulated. It is something that all coaches should be aware of (see Chapter 10).

Risk of injury is a further consideration, particularly for those who compete regularly at a senior level. A serious injury may render a lifter unable to work, and few powerlifters are fortunate enough to have an insurance plan that would cover complete loss of earnings and any rehabilitation that may be required.

Female lifters have a further consideration. If they make powerlifting their career, which can easily span ten years, they may have to decide to delay having a family or choose to compete for a few years, establish themselves and take time out to have a family. They must then balance motherhood and competing. This can be achieved successfully, but the workload increases dramatically and can place extra strain on both the lifter's body and their support network.

For both male and female lifters a sporting pathway can inhibit career advancement since an employer may feel that all the passion, drive and time devoted to the sport is likely to dilute their commitment to their profession.

Even a professional coach who is also a lifter in their own right will face a conflict of interest between their own lifting and their 'day job' and, on occasions, it may be difficult to remain focused on the athlete they are being paid to coach. At some point the coach must decide if they are predominantly a coach or a lifter. If they continue to play a dual role, it can be deemed unethical if they compete against any athlete they have coached or supported to the platform.

To compete or not to compete is a personal decision. For some talented lifters, competing can cause a lot of stress and worry and may not be worthwhile. Others thrive on the feeling of escapism that results from training and will enjoy developing a healthy lifestyle and a new social circle. The pros and cons should be carefully considered and each lifter must create a lifestyle balance according to their circumstances, their personal needs and the needs of those around them.

CHAPTER 8

COACH-LED SERVICES

There are many support services available to help powerlifters achieve their goals, be they novices or elite athletes. Most lifters start with massage and basic nutritional advice which they have to source and fund themselves since powerlifting is not an Olympic funded sport and relies heavily on private sponsorship. Paralympic powerlifters and weightlifters attached to a British team, on the other hand, have access to a full range of service providers, including sports scientists, doctors, physiotherapists, psychologists, nutritionists and masseurs as part of a funded world-class training programme.

This chapter discusses some of the key services that lifters are likely to require as they strive to achieve their end goals. While novice lifters will not have a sporting support package around them, they will benefit from knowing which services are available. For advice on the types of services available and where to access them, contact the relevant national federation. It should be stated here that this chapter does not intend to provide a detailed discussion of sports science which incorporates areas of physiology, psychology, biomechanics, nutrition, sports technology, performance analysis and performance lifestyle. Sports science is very well established within some of the larger Olympic and Paralympic sports, although this is not currently the case within IPF powerlifting where most athletes are self-funded.

All the services play an important role and can be called into play either singly or in combination, depending on the issue that needs to be addressed. A coach should have a working knowledge of the services available and know when to bring in specialist providers to respond to or pre-empt issues and challenges. This can become something of a balancing act.

The Role of Nutrition

The nutritional aspect of a lifter's daily life and competition preparation is imperative in promoting and maintaining good health and enhancing sporting performance. A sports nutritionist is able to translate scientific data about an athlete's body composition (for example, their metabolic measurements) into a tailored and practical nutritional plan, which will consider the lifter's training regime and will be designed to ensure that sufficient food is taken on board to achieve the desired training output and to enhance recovery afterwards. The nutritionist will advise on good food choices, taking into account the athlete's preferences and possibly introducing new foods into their diet.

Accredited sports nutritionists can advise on the optimal body weight class that a lifter should be placed in at any given point during their sporting career. For example, they can assess that an athlete with a high metabolic rate is unlikely to move up a weight class and vice versa. They have expert knowledge of the best athlete-specific body composition and can identify the most favourable combinations of food groups for use as fuel in training or for storage by the body for muscle repair, all of which will correlate with the lifter's training output.

Nutritionists can educate the lifter to opt for informed food choices and align these to lifestyle commitments, cultural requirements, gender, budget and any underlying health issues.

They can help them improve their understanding of food supplements and hydration levels, work with them on pre- and post-competition weigh-in strategies and design dietary plans for international travel and competitions.

An athlete's ability to access the services of a nutritionist is largely dictated by available funding. Since IPF powerlifting is not currently a funded sport even athletes selected to represent Great Britain may not have the opportunity to work with a nutritionist on an individual basis. Paralympic powerlifters, however, do currently receive funding and so will be able to access the services of a nutritionist far more easily.

Body weight class food diary

A key question for all powerlifters is: 'Which body weight class am I best suited to?' This issue will be subject to ongoing review and analysis during a lifter's career, as an individual may compete across as many as three different body weight classes over a few years. To illustrate, a lifter may start with little muscle mass so will initially lift relatively light weights. As they continue to train and build muscle, they are likely to reduce fat and measure less on particular body parts, such as the waist, upper thighs and arms. Since muscle weighs more than fat, they will weigh more on the scales although they will have a far better body composition.

Often, new lifters find themselves between body weight classes and are unsure if they should move down a weight class or move up to the one above. A novice powerlifter would be wise to lift at their natural body weight and adopt a healthy eating plan. They should then record what they eat and reassess this as their lifting technique improves and body composition begins to change.

All lifters will benefit from keeping a food diary and monitoring their body weight on a weekly basis. The diary will record and reveal a great deal of valuable information about what is being consumed each day and each week, including:

- The exact number of calories.
- Hidden fats, fructose and empty calories such as alcohol units.
- Eating patterns and fads over training days and non-training days.
- Combinations of protein and carbohydrates.
- Fluids, iron, vitamins, minerals and the more intense levels of supplements such as branch chain amino acids and creatine (powder formulation of protein).

The diary will also reveal differences in intake between training days lifting heavy tonnage compared with days lifting less weight when the focus is more on technique.

The more data that is recorded, the easier it becomes to identify small changes that could make a big difference. It is not uncommon for lifters to consume too much protein in relation to carbohydrates, in the belief that they must build muscle above all else in order to be able to lift the weights. What they should also remember is that carbohydrates provide the vital energy that fuels their muscle body systems that enable them to undertake training programmes in the first place, so it is important to achieve a balance. Other lifters may cut their fat intake to below recommended amounts in order to become leaner and because they understand that, unlike muscle, fat is less functional for their perceived goal. This can be dangerous because too little fat in the diet can result in loss of essential fatty acids and fat soluble vitamins that the body needs to survive. Food diary entries will soon reveal deficiencies and potential areas of risk, enabling corrective action to be taken. At the end of the day athletes should understand that they need to feed the whole body, not just the muscle.

It is important to recognize that, for a food diary to work, all the foods consumed must be recorded. This includes 'forgotten' items that never reach the dinner plate, for instance a bite of a friend's burger or ingredients nibbled whilst preparing a meal. In the beginning it is also helpful to record how food is cooked, for example frying or grilling. All foods have calorific value and once eaten contribute to the daily food intake total.

The training diary is an excellent tool for setting healthy, manageable body weight goals and helping the lifter stay on track. It also helps to identify the ideal training and competition body weights, which can differ by up to 4kg. No two lifters have the same body composition but, by monitoring body weight changes and food and fluid intake, a more scientific approach to weight management and resulting performance can be taken. For instance, a lifter can more easily establish if they should increase or decrease calorie intake a few days before a competition, and an appropriate plan for nutritional intervention can be put in place. This might involve reducing portion sizes and altering eating times over a period of a few days or it may be a plan that will be carried out over four to six weeks. Irrespective of weight loss or gain, any nutritional intervention must be implemented within healthy guidelines, and great caution should be exercised when considering the use of diuretics to aid weight reduction, as the majority of these products are on the banned list.

Each coach takes a different approach to helping their athlete achieve their desired competition weight. For example, some are happy for their athletes to be 2kg above competition weight during training and will build a plan to reduce the weight four weeks before the competition.

Others prefer their athlete to train at competition weight. The key is to know exactly when the athlete is at risk of losing strength by losing weight. This will be different for each lifter.

If a lifter is unable to consult a sport-specific nutritionist they could talk to their local heath adviser or consider attending an educational course to learn about the breakdown of food groups, the optimal times to eat pre- and post-training and post-weigh-in at competitions, the best type of recovery foods and the most appropriate form in which to take food onboard relative to the circumstances. Alternatively, their gym proprietor may know of a reputable coach who could recommend some good literature or a service provider with whom they have links. Their lifting federation may also have a contact that would be willing to look at a food diary or offer advice. An alternative option could be to contact a local university that offers degrees in nutrition and ask if a third-year student would be willing to provide some supervised advice. It may even be possible for a lifter to trade their professional skills with those of the nutritionist.

Ascertaining body composition

A suitably accredited nutritionist is likely to ask for a food diary to be completed and they will specify how they want the information to be captured. To help them gain a full picture they will probably want to ascertain the lifter's start-

FOOD FOR THOUGHT

- Choose a variety of food groups to give the body everything it needs for muscle growth and repair; include fats as the internal organs need these to function.
- Do not cut out a food group completely unless advised to do so on medical grounds by a qualified health professional.
- Think about portion sizes, empty calories, eating times, food combinations and preparation.
- Maintain a food diary.
- Learn to read food labels.
- Be very clear about where any supplements used are produced and what they may contain.
- Think ahead if travelling or working long hours and plan accordingly.

ing body weight and body composition. To do this they will need to identify the lifter's muscle-to-fat ratio which will involve the use of various tests and measurements.

The skin fold test, also known as the pinch test, is one of the more easily available. Here, callipers are used to take measurements on target areas around the body, and the data is kept for comparison over time. This test is directed at the thickness of the subcutaneous fat layer covering the body, and an equation comparing height, body weight and girth of the bones is used to estimate the lifter's percentage of body fat. Care must be taken to ensure that the same callipers are used on the same test sites each time the test is performed to ensure accurate monitoring.

There are various ways to calculate the body's fat-to-muscle ratio with some accuracy. However, the most commonly used method, the body mass index (BMI), is not a good predictor for the majority of powerlifters. The BMI is an index reference chart that draws on data from a huge population of comparative individuals. Focusing on the best possible predicted body mass by analyzing an individual's height and body weight, it is based on the relative law of averages. However, powerlifters do not fit within the 'normal' range since they weigh more than the average person, having developed far more muscle mass while aiming to reduce the percentage of body fat. Based on the BMI index they are frequently informed that they are obese.

Top athletes use a variety of methods to ascertain body composition as accurately as possible. These include body scans, ultrasound, electrodes and bioimpedance. The aim is to identify body fat percentage, bone density and total body water and potassium content. This can be an expensive process, although with some creativity it may be possible to reduce the cost. For example, some university sports science departments have the necessary equipment and expertise and may be willing to do the scan for a nominal charge in return for using the data collected for their research. If the lifter is to represent Great Britain it may be possible to negotiate a reduced fee with the equipment owners who could also take advantage of PR opportunities.

Accepting the continuing debates as to the accuracy and consistency of the above methods, it should be recognized that all offer a baseline normative that will set the foundations for long-term athlete-specific data. The key is to record and interoperate any data correctly and then work with the results to achieve the right food intake for the lifter and to assign them to the appropriate body weight class.

The use of supplements

There will be occasions when a lifter will be rushed or have other constraints on their time and may feel unable to consume and digest the amount of calories required in a solid meal format. At such times supplements may be introduced and the nutritionist can advise accordingly. Supplements include vitamins, minerals, herbs, meal replacements, fortified snacks that complement a meal and concentrated protein products such as branch chain amino acids. Snack bars also count as supplements and there are many sport types available; some have a high protein content while others are carbohydrate and sugar-based. There is also a vast range of carbohydrate and protein shakes and drinks available. All are designed to enhance the nutritional content of the eating plan.

Supplements should be used wisely and must not be considered as an alternative to poor food choices. They can be expensive and should be well vetted since, depending on where they are made or purchased, there may be a link to banned substances. The nutritionist will be able to advise on the correct type to be used as part of the nutrition plan.

All eating plans should be athlete-specific. However, certain groups of individuals will need to take different variables into account. For example, vegans or athletes with medical disorders such as diabetes or Crohn's disease will need to include good quality proteins from various sources, while those with a dairy intolerance will need to source calcium-rich alternatives.

Any nutritional plan for a female athlete must take their menstrual cycle into account. The diet should not produce deficits linked to osteoporosis or side effects leading to menstrual dysfunction. Iron and hormone levels should also be monitored as long-term absence of periods can cause loss of bone density which cannot be recovered.

If an athlete has any type of medical condition or special dietary requirements, they should speak to their general practitioner before any nutritional intervention is introduced.

Nutrition and international travel

When travelling to overseas training camps, squads and competitions it is vital for an athlete to have the correct foods available at the right time to facilitate maximum performance. This requires careful research into the food types available at the ultimate destination and planning accordingly. In some countries the diet is rice-based so an athlete needs to ensure that enough protein is available, for example by bringing their own high protein shakes and then reducing their rice intake at their destination. Sufficient food and supplements should be taken for the duration of the whole trip, allowing for any delays. This may include snacks and prepared food and unopened bottled water and sports drinks, usually shipped as cargo. It is important to avoid overeating or going for long periods without food as this may result in nutritional deficiency.

A nutritionist will consider international time zones and develop a plan to manage food intake accordingly. Supplements will help here, for example, eating protein bars on the plane instead of the flight meals provided. For long-haul journeys, the nutritionist will work out what type of snacks should be eaten within each time zone, thus helping the lifter acclimatize to their final destination. In practice, this could mean eating a snack when other passengers are sleeping.

NUTRITION AND TRAVEL

Athletes should:

- Have a well thought out and rehearsed nutrition plan and stick to it; post-event, they should revise and re-plan.
- Carefully research which foods can be taken into the country they are travelling to, and note and plan around any restrictions.
- Not rely on being able to buy all their food abroad as ingredients may vary.
- Be aware that different countries have different policies on the temperature at which food is cooked and refrigerated.
- Accept that they may experience stomach upsets until they have adapted to the local cuisine.
- Avoid local cuisine before competing, for the same reason as above.

In summary, a good nutritional adviser will understand elite sport and performance and be able to provide information and feedback in a clear and practical way. In turn, the athlete should be prepared to learn about making appropriate choices from the different food groups.

The Role of Physiotherapy

Massage

The more powerlifters push their bodies to the limit and force muscle adaptation to increase strength and power while maintaining flexibility, the more they will benefit from exploring the various methods that help with recovery and replenishment. There are various types of physical therapy available so it is important that the correct approach and technique is matched to the athlete's needs.

Massage has been shown to benefit many athletes and can be used to support general maintenance, enhance injury recovery or alleviate stress. Soft tissue massage, often known as Swedish massage, manipulates the muscles and tendons. This type of massage is often conducted in a relaxed setting, with soft music playing to combat both mental and physical fatigue. It can be extremely beneficial post-competition, but it is not advised pre-competition as the lifter can become too relaxed to achieve maximum output.

Sports massage focuses on deep tissue work and the use of trigger points and is much firmer than a general massage. It can help reduce spasms and discomfort in both injured tissue and the muscles which work to compensate an injury site. It is frequently used to ease trouble spots such as knots in the belly of the muscle which are usually caused by poor technique or previous injuries. It also helps to promote blood flow around the body and remove some of the metabolic by-products produced by intensive exercise. In turn this supports recovery between training sessions and can help with injury prevention.

PNF (Proprioceptive Neuromuscular Facilitation) is a sports massage technique (used by other therapists too) that helps improve muscle flexibility and range of motion. It involves stretching the body part, letting it relax, and then stretching it again. It is extremely useful for powerlifters who frequently become very tight in the hamstrings, trapezius and lower lumbar region.

A masseur can offer rehabilitation massage and often works alongside a physiotherapist to help manage injury recovery. As with all service providers, it is important that they work with other professionals and that they are acutely aware of when to hand over to a different service. For example, after conducting an initial consultation, a good masseur will know if massage would be the correct treatment in relation to the symptoms and feedback being presented by the athlete. Consequently, they will know when to advise the athlete to see their GP or a physiotherapist as opposed to beginning a treatment package themselves.

Prophylactic physiotherapy

If a lifter is experiencing pain, recovering from surgery, has developed a muscle imbalance which impedes performance or is likely to incur further injury or experience injury re-occurrence, they are likely to be referred to a specialist sports physiotherapist. Physiotherapists offer prophylactic care, defined as the management of injuries through prevention rehabilitation. Specifically, they work with the neuromuscular systems to aid recovery, reduce pain, improve functionality, regain full range of movement, including the power output of the limb and restructure muscle imbalance and muscle tone, all promoting a high level of physical health. They often work with a full medical team and know who to collaborate with and when to get the best outcome for the athlete. Therapists can work alongside coaches to gain an understanding of the muscles that need to be recruited and the posture that should be held when performing a particular exercise.

Physiotherapists draw on several methods and skills to aid lifters. These may include electrotherapy, to stimulate muscle fibres and blood flow and acupuncture, which has been found to help in the treatment of injuries and the relief of muscle pain. They have an intense knowledge of surgery and a solid appreciation of when this should or should not be undertaken. They have an up-to-date understanding of strapping and support to help with training, injury prevention and rehabilitation.

The Role of Psychology

The discipline of sports and exercise psychology plays an integral role within powerlifting as it focuses on how the brain and psyche work in sporting situations. As with all the sciences it has many complexities, and therefore this chapter can only provide an overview of how it may be used within the sport.

A good practitioner can help with a multitude of performance factors yet will also know when

WHAT THE EYE CANNOT SEE – CASE STUDY

For many years I coached a world-class bench presser. Over time, his muscle bulk intensified and he became restricted in the shoulder girth. As a result, he felt that his chest was about to tear when he brought the bar down. Although he was able to create a huge arch position from which to press, the arch elongated and flattened when the bar moved off the chest. At world-class level, when an athlete is lifting to their 1 rep max (the heaviest weight they can lift in any particular exercise), this can cause them to sway under load or push the bar further than necessary. This can make the difference between a good lift and a fail. The reason for this is that, although the arch has become depressed, the bar still has to continue on its pathway but now must travel further to compensate for the slightly flattened arch. In turn this can make it difficult for a lifter with a weak lock-out as it may appear to the referees that the press has not been fully locked. It could also appear that the bar creates a double movement at the latter stage of the ascent. Alternatively, a referee may consider the arch collapsing as a change of elected body movement between the start and finish of the lift. Any of these aspects would result in a failure, although this may not become apparent until the third lift when the weight has been increased to the maximum.

This particular case was not easy for me to navigate alone so I called in a physiotherapist who viewed video footage of the athlete's lifts and came to the gym to see him in action. It transpired that, while the gluteus maximus was fully contracting, the gluteus medius was barely firing at all and the insertion into the left rotator cuff was significantly weaker than the right side. In addition, it transpired that the top three vertebrae in the spine had little to no flexibility. Although the misalignment of the bar had been evident through tracking and analysis of its pathway, none of the physical issues had been apparent to the naked eye. It was the physiotherapist who diagnosed the weaknesses in the muscles and skeletal rigidity and prescribed a range of exercises. These were carried out three times a day for eight weeks at which point a reduced number of more intense exercises was incorporated into the warm-up routine for both the squat and bench press.

By strengthening the gluteus medius the lifter was able to push the arch up from the bottom half of the body and maintain this position rather than just perching from the scapular. The sternum was able to push up 1.5cm higher than previously and the entire rotary cuff was strengthened and balanced. This took three months to achieve and resulted in an improved body shape under load and the lifter going on to gain a silver medal at the Commonwealth Games, clearly demonstrating the value of the physiotherapist's intervention.

to hand over to, and work with, other service providers and consultants. This could be when a disorder is identified. For example, a sports psychologist may identify that an athlete has issues with anger management. The sport may be a controlled outlet for their anger but, in itself, is not the cure and a psychologist would know when and how to set up an appropriate support network for the athlete. Similarly, a psychologist may identify an underlying eating disorder and would set up a support network which might involve contacting the athlete's GP and bringing in a clinical psychologist who specializes in specific eating disorders.

Coaches should be aware that individuals who are overly concerned with their body weight and image may be attracted to powerlifting or weightlifting. As these are both weight class sports, they provide an avenue for athletes to justifiably and actively control and record their body weight without demonstrating any obvious cause for concern. The key is to know what is normal behaviour for the sport and to be able to spot when behaviour becomes obsessive. A good coach should know when to involve a sports psychologist to assist. The right support can help athletes to understand that good dietary practice will lead to a healthy functional body shape and corresponding weight.

Performance output can be enhanced via different aspects of sport psychology, which in turn help with issues such as focus, anger management or goal-setting. Athletes can work on a few components at once or they may prefer to focus on one aspect which they regard as the biggest inhibitor to performance and then move on to tackle other components. This said, the practitioner is always working to foster self-reliance, aiming to pass on the skills required to the athlete and coach, thus making themselves redundant. This is imperative as the lifter is the only person who can go onto the platform and perform the lifts. Everyone else is relegated to the sidelines.

Sports psychology has many different tools that can be used either singly or in combination to achieve the desired outcomes. Coaches and athletes should develop an awareness of when and how sports psychology can help so that they are better placed to identify problems when they arise and know where to go for advice and possible assistance.

Focus

A well-documented psychological factor in powerlifting is the lifter's ability to focus during competition, especially when they are about to lift a maximum weight. Sports psychologists have a deep knowledge of the concepts of focus, attention and concentration and spend years developing strategies for different personality types in order to help individuals increase the quality and control of their concentration span. Focus is taken to mean the ability to concentrate effectively on an imminent assignment, or the most prevalent factor in a given situation, to the exclusion of any other distractions.

This intensive concentration is immensely helpful for lifters during the warm-up phase of a competition, which is likely to be one of the few times when they will share a lifting platform alongside peers or champions. This can be distracting and may cause a lifter to lose concentration and momentarily neglect the attention to detail that they should be paying to their own lifting technique. For example, in the squat they may not go low enough on the last warm-up so if they repeat this mistake in their first lifting attempt, they may easily fail.

The key is to learn to focus on tangible things such as where the bar sits in the racks. With practice distractions such as sharing a warm-up platform with a world champion will blend into the background and the detail of the job in hand will become the central focus. As a lifter becomes more proficient at this psychological skill they can switch their attention and relax the mind between lifts and return to acute focus when required.

Goal-setting

Goal-setting is another well-known psychological technique used in powerlifting to help lifters achieve their overall objectives. By deciding which body weight class a lifter should compete in and writing a training programme for them, a coach is setting goals and incremental targets as part of an overall lifting plan. Within this plan one goal might be to increase the bench press by 2.5kg in eight weeks and lose 1kg in body weight in the same time frame.

There are various types of goals within the realm of sport. One of the most popular is known as an 'outcome' or 'end' goal (the terms are interchangeable). Within a sporting context, this kind of goal is linked to performing better than someone else, for example by winning a medal or competition. To achieve an outcome goal, underlying 'performance goals' are set, which concentrate on the individual lifter's performance so they are not dependent on what other competitors may achieve. The outcome is measured by comparing the performance result against a previous result the athlete has already achieved. To illustrate, if a powerlifter gained a 90kg bench press and seven white lights in January, the performance goal could be to gain 95kg and eight white lights by April. Obtaining this goal will increase the lifter's total, helping them to achieve their outcome goal of winning a medal.

Both the coach and the lifter can benefit greatly from seeking help in agreeing goals, identifying and understanding the process for achieving these and deciding the responsibility each should take along the way. As an example, the coach and lifter's outcome goal may appear to be the same: to win at a major competition. However, there might be disagreement on the timeline or the route required to achieve this goal. The lifter may wish to win both the European championships and the best lifter award at the British championships to be held six weeks before. The coach might think it unrealistic to obtain both goals as the best lifter award would require the lifter to give 100 per cent effort on each discipline. By over-reaching at the British championships they could risk not achieving the overall goal of winning the European title.

The coach might therefore want to set different targets for the British championships such as gaining a Personal Best lift on the squat (an outcome goal) or trying a slightly different stance on the deadlift (a process goal), while aiming to obtain a minimum of seven out of nine lifts. From a coaching perspective this would work as a transition route to align the lifter with the overall goal of becoming European champion. This would be achieved by setting three different underlying targets: the weight lifted for the squat; improved technique enabling the lifter to lift the weight more comfortably on the deadlift; holding mental focus by gaining seven out of nine lifts. This coaching strategy would be aimed at preventing over-training and poor recovery for the impending European championships.

Conversely, the lifter may consider any plan that does not focus on gaining the best lifter award as a reduced outcome goal and an indication that the coach does not believe they have the potential to win the Europeans. In turn this could affect the lifter's self-confidence and/or erode the coach/lifter relationship.

A sports psychologist would be able to unpick why the lifter has attached so much significance to the best lifter award and help to identify the lifter's long-term goals, which could well mean taking a year out to concentrate on the best lifter award on home ground. They would also be able to help the coach and lifter merge their ideas and build goal attainment strategies that both are happy to work to and take responsibility for.

Whatever the labels, a well-crafted plan of how to get from A to B is essential. The key is to know when to focus on a particular type of goal and not over-focus on the final outcome. Coaches and lifters alike have aspirations and dreams; goal setting offers an approach to turn an aspiration into a workable pathway that enables the individual to reach their true potential.

Sports and exercise psychologists can offer expert further advice on many more components such as how to deal with anxiety under pressure, not taking responsibility for performance, the use of mental imagery, burn-out, low self-esteem and a multitude of other aspects to improve mental preparation and enhance performance output.

Athletes often self-refer in order to access the services of a sport psychologist. If they are linked to a funded programme or sponsor they may be able to access the service as part of the performance package that has been put in place for them.

CHAPTER 9

THE PHASES OF A COMPETITION

Before the Competition

Technical meeting

Prior to the competition a technical meeting will be held by the appointed technical committee, consisting of event officials and their representatives. All countries/teams will be invited to attend via their appointed team manager or official team representative. The aim of all technical meetings is to ensure fair play from all points of view. The overall objective is to ensure that the rules for the sport are suitably and consistently adhered to. The format for the meeting will be sent out to all concerned prior to the event, and generally covers the following:

- A roll call of each country (for an international event).
- A list of the pre-registered body weights in each class for the competition.
- The chairperson reads out the names of the athletes registered in each body weight class and asks their representative to confirm that their name and date of birth are as shown in their passport and that they will be lifting within the registered body weight class. Any discrepancies must be declared and corrected at this point, noting there is likely to be a forfeit to be paid for any change made to any body weight class. All changes that will affect the order of the competition or state of play will be sent out by the technical committee to all involved prior to the competition.
- The competition schedule is clearly defined and explained.
- Any clarification of the rules and protocols

and any other business are discussed at this point.

Order of competition

The competition schedule is sent out in advance and should be checked carefully as the order of lifting can vary from one event to another. For instance, in one competition all the ladies may lift first and the men afterwards, both groups lifting in ascending body weight order. In another, the men and ladies may alternate, for example ladies' lightest, men's lightest, ladies' next weight class, men's next weight class and so on.

Personal apparel

Lifters should familiarize themselves with the correct personal apparel before a competition. A rule that many forget is that all kit should be clean and of a suitable quality; this is subject to the referee's interpretation. If a lifter is found to be wearing any unauthorized kit they will be eliminated from the competition and any total achieved will be disqualified.

On the Day of Competition

To host a powerlifting competition a venue should be able to provide sufficient space for a lifting platform, ideally with a reinforced floor, a separate warm-up room and an area to accommodate an audience. There should also be space, preferably separate rooms, to facilitate the weigh-in and drug testing processes. Such venues tend to be colleges, schools, gyms and sports clubs. For international events hotels and conference centres are often used.

On competition day at British Championships and above, a lifter signs in on entry to the venue and has their name ticked off the lifting register. At this point they must also complete and sign a drug testing form and be prepared to be tested for banned substances under in-competition rules or they will not be allowed to compete. It is worth noting here that it is possible for a lifter to be tested if they have signed in but are subsequently unable to compete. Lifters are subject to competition testing for up to 12 hours before the event. (This is different to out-of-competition testing where, while the test is the same, the testers are looking for slightly different ratios.) Athletes won't know if the testers are present until they come to lift.

On arrival, it is a good idea to confirm that the order of the day's events is the same as advertised. At local competitions the organizers may bring forward a weigh-in slot if there are fewer lifters than expected and if all relevant parties agree. At international championships, where European and World records are likely to be attempted, the schedule would remain as advertised.

To be fully prepared lifters should arrive early and ascertain their rack heights on the actual competition squat and bench press racks, noting that these may be different from those in the warm-up room.

Kit check

Kit check begins before the weigh-in (where the lifter mounts the scales and their body weight is recorded) but may continue during the 1½-hour weigh-in process. All kit to be worn on the lifting platform must be checked by qualified referees. In a divisional competition this may be carried out by a single referee, while at national level and above there may be five referees or more. Each item of kit must be inspected to ensure that it corresponds to the rules and be ticked off the kit check list. For example, all wrist and knee wraps must be measured to ensure they are the correct length. If they are too long the lifter must decide if they will use wraps at all,

cut them down to the correct length or try to borrow a pair of the correct specification.

During the competition a designated technical officer will be based in the warm-up room to ensure that no lifter is wearing kit that has not been checked in. A lifter can be prevented from going out for an attempt if something appears to be incorrect. The time taken to ratify this will be deducted from the lifter's 60-second lifting time. This can be a big distraction for the lifter and may have a negative impact on performance, so it is very important to make the correct kit choices within the context of the rules.

Weigh-in lot order

A lot draw is undertaken prior to the weigh-in and each lifter in the competition is randomly assigned a number which is theirs for the duration of the competition. The lifters are weighed in ascending order according to the lot order numbers. For example, if one lifter has the number 22 and another has 3, number 3 will be called to the scales first.

Coaches should note that if two lifters wish to lift the same weight in the same lifting round, the lifter with the lower lot number will lift first. On last lifts this can be a disadvantage as the lifter with the higher lot order will be able to see if the lifter with the lower lot number lmade a successful attempt or not. This gives them the opportunity to stay at the same weight if the attempt failed or go up if it was successful. Either way, they have an advantage over the lifter with the lower lot order. On the other hand the lifter with the lower lot order who can weigh in first will have more time to prepare themselves before lifting commences.

Weigh-in

After completing their registration forms the lifter must proceed to the weigh-in area where there will be a list of the athletes' names, country (or club) and allocated lot numbers. At all ratified events the weigh-in commences two hours before the competition starts and lasts for 1½ hours. Lifters are advised to be ready and waiting five minutes beforehand, regardless of lot order. If a lifter's name is called and they are not present, the next lifter on the list is called and the first named lifter will then have to wait until all the others have been called to mount the scales.

If a lifter is overweight, they will be given the opportunity to 'make weight' as many times as necessary. However, this can only be done once all the other lifters have been weighed in and only within the time constraints of the 1½ hours weigh-in timeframe. If other lifters have not made weight this should also be taken into consideration. There are various ways to make weight including visiting the bathroom, taking a brisk walk in a full track suit and wiping off perspiration afterwards. It has been known for male athletes to shave the hair on their head and arms.

When a lifter is called to the scales they will be asked to declare their rack heights and their opening lifts. At this point they must also provide proof of federation membership and proof of identity, including age. At IPC Powerlifting events a lifting licence will also be requested.

Lifters usually mount the scales in their under-wear, although they can choose to remove all attire, which is quite usual for qualifying events. Currently, bench press athletes with a lower limb amputation should be weighed without their prosthesis and additions will be made to their body weight accordingly (see lifting federa-tion rules). The weigh-in takes place in the pres-ence of two referees of the same gender as the lifter. The lifter and referees must check and agree that the weight has been registered and displayed on the scales. When all concerned are in consensus, the lifter and the referee sign to confirm the actual body weight and the opening attempts of each discipline in the competition and the corresponding rack heights.

The lifter is then given attempt cards which show their name, country or club, weight class and body weight. Three attempts are permitted for the squat and bench press and five for the deadlift. The lifter may change their declared first attempt up to five minutes before the start of the round. Once they have completed a lift, they have 60 seconds to declare their next attempt. The coach or lifter then presents the attempt card to the designated referee who must co-sign this to confirm they have received the request of the next attempt.

All of the details given in at the weigh-in are transmitted to a scoreboard located next to the lifting platform, enabling the audience and coaches to follow the competition. There will also be smaller versions of the scoreboard in the warm-up room to save coaches having to move back and forth.

Taking food on board

A lifter may have to wait as long as 1 hour 45 minutes before lifting, if they were first to weigh in, or as little as 25 minutes if they were last or had to re-weigh. All lifters should prepare to be weighed-in last and make provision for taking on board the best types of foods. Every lifter will differ, but the basic rule is to take on fluids and food that give slow release energy, for example drinks or sugars to help with energy dips throughout the competition, all of which should be digested with relative ease. The lifter should avoid becoming dehydrated, and if dehy-dration has taken place in order to make weight they should take action swiftly to replenish the body. By the same token, lifters do not want to take on too much fluid too quickly, as it is chal-lenging not to mention time-consuming to get in and out of the lifting suits in order to take a comfort break.

Warming-up

The warm-up process typically involves stretch-ing, performing some lifts without lifting apparel, putting on the lifting apparel and lifting weights progressively by reducing the reps and increas-ing the weight towards their competition one rep max. While each lifter knows how long it takes to warm up, it is a good idea to build in at least another 15 minutes to accommodate any unforeseen circumstances.

Lifters are not usually permitted to warm up in the warm-up room until the previous group of competitors is on their last round. Ideally, there will be enough weights and racks for all nations and competitors, although this may be something of a luxury and lifters should expect to share. It is sensible for lifters to get to the warm-up room early, identify the set of racks they would prefer, which is a personal choice, and try to 'claim' it before anyone else. If the lifter has good relationships with other nations or lifters it is worth asking if they are happy to share.

Approximately fifteen minutes before the start of the competition the lifters who are about to compete are called to the platform and presented to the audience. As their name is called out each lifter takes a step forward and a short testament to their achievements is read out. The referees are also introduced to the audience. This process can take up to ten minutes and cause a break in the warm-ups so this should be factored in to the lifter's preparation time.

Following the presentation to the audience, the last call for any changes to the opening lift is made which, as previously stated, is five minutes before lifting commences. Coaches must take this into consideration to ensure that the lifter is able to complete their warm-up before going onto the platform. Lifters and coaches must be clear which clock at the venue is being used as the official competition clock, and then synchronize their watches to this. Being just one minute out can make the difference between a lifter putting in a credible performance or failing.

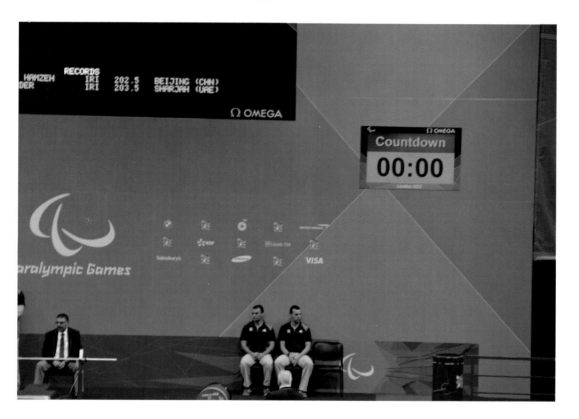

The competition clock, Paralympic Games bench press, London 2012.

TIME TACTICS – CASE STUDY

I was coaching at a championships in Europe where it was extremely warm. The venue resembled a marquee, which made the conditions very humid. One lifter I was coaching at the time became very lethargic and started to perspire profusely. Meanwhile, another of my lifters was thriving in the heat. At the same time I noticed that the Australian team were enjoying the heat and doing very well in their warm-ups while some of the other European countries seemed to be struggling.

I made the decision to reduce both the warm-up and opening lifts for my struggling lifter by 10kg. My last opportunity to do this was five minutes before the start of the round so I had to pick my moment carefully and ensure that I was referring to the correct clock.

Earlier that morning I had discovered there were three main clocks in the venue: one belonged to the venue while the other two had been provided by the competition organizers. However, there was a discrepancy of two minutes between the clock in the warm-up room and the clock on the main scoreboard so I asked the chief referee which of the clocks was to be used as the competition clock. It was the scoreboard clock.

I reduced my lifter's attempts accordingly, and coaches from other nations did the same for their lifters. However, two coaches were caught out and their change of attempt was not accepted as they were too late. Consequently neither of their lifters had a very good competition as all their efforts went into gaining the first lift which under the conditions was too draining for them.

By forward planning and reducing the first attempt using the correct clock, I was pleased that the lifter I was coaching placed higher than the two lifters who had to stay with their original opening lifts. In normal circumstances these individuals were likely to have placed higher and may even have medalled.

The round system

When the competition commences the bar is loaded to the lightest weight and the announcers state the lifter's name (and country, if international) and the weight to be attempted. Once the referees are in place and the chief referee is satisfied that all is correct the latter will say 'Bar is loaded'. The clock then starts, giving the lifter 60 seconds to commence the lift. The lifter steps onto the platform, sets up the lift and makes the attempt between the referee's signals. Irrespective of a good or bad attempt, they must leave the platform and declare their next attempt within sixty seconds.

Once the competition is under way, lifting is conducted following what is known as a round system. Here, the lifter who is to attempt the lightest weight goes first. If there is more than one lifter attempting the same weight, the lifts take place in ascending order of lot number. The bar is then loaded in incremental weights until the last person in the group has performed their first attempt. For instance the opening weight of the squat could be 180kg and could finish at 270kg with the last lifter's first attempt. When each lifter has made their first attempt this is the end of Round 1. The bar is then reduced to the starting weight of the first lifter in Round 2 and the process is repeated in the second and third rounds.

If there are more than ten lifters they will be divided into alphabetical groups. Hence there could be a Group A and a Group B. Group B would compete first, followed by Group A.

Again, the lifting takes place in ascending order with the lighter weights going first.

The weight on the bar is never reduced once the round has started even if there has been a mistake during the loading phase. Therefore, if the bar was loaded at 170kg instead of 175kg and the lifter gained a successful lift, they could accept the lift and move on to their next attempt in the following round. Alternatively, they could request another attempt at the correct weight which would take place at the end of the round. However, if that attempt was unsuccessful they could not then reclaim the first successful attempt. Alternatively, if they failed the 175kg they could request another attempt at 170kg to take place at the end of the round.

Occasionally, the bar is mis-loaded at a heavier weight – I have witnessed a bar being overloaded by 15kg, which was 5kg more than the lifter's current Personal Best. The lifter gained a successful lift with a weight they had been failing for the previous twelve months and went on to achieve a lifetime's best total. They put this achievement down to not knowing what was on the bar and being utterly determined not to fail.

Protests

If a lifter or coach is unhappy with a referee's decision they have the right to put in a protest and must do so by submitting the correct forms within sixty seconds of the disputed lift being completed. Currently, a fee of US $100 is payable to the competition's lifting federation, irrespective of where the competition is being held. If the decision is overturned the lift cannot be given back and the lifter will be given the opportunity to take the lift again at the end of the round. If the decision is upheld the fee will be retained by the federation. (It has been known for a coach to put in a tactical protest against another lifter, quite expecting to lose, the objective being to slow down the proceedings to give their lifter a little more rest time between lifts.)

Record attempts

Record attempts cover many categories, such as British, European, Commonwealth, World and Paralympic. There are also age categories for records, such as junior (up to age 24), Masters 1 (over 40 years) and Masters 2 (over 50 years) and so on. Each record attempt must be claimed at the appropriate level of competition. To illustrate, it would not be possible to claim a national record at a World championships – it would have to be at least a European record granted with the permission of the Chief Referee or Head of Jury. It would, however, be acceptable to take a World record at a European championships. Regardless of the circumstances, it is the lifter's responsibility to fill in the relevant forms and claim the record in their name.

Coaches and lifters must be very clear about their goals and targets and the expectations of sponsors. A lifter attached to a world-class performance programme is dependent on medals, not records to secure their funding, while an independent athlete may be very happy to obtain a record over a medal place.

Competition tactics

There is a fundamental difference between the last round of a bench press-only competition and the deadlift as the last lift in a full three-lift powerlifting competition. The subtotal in a bench press-only competition is derived from the first and second lifts. The subtotal in a three-lift competition (squat, bench press and deadlift) is the final total of the squat and the final total of the bench press combined. The competition is won on three lifts. Any records achieved at a fourth attempt do not go towards the sub-total.

Tactics come into play throughout the competition. A coach needs to know which lifts their lifter can excel at and which lifts best suit the opponents and make tactical decisions accordingly. To illustrate, if a lifter is an excellent squatter and can place themselves 25kg ahead, but an opponent has a superb deadlift (the last of the three powerlifting lifts) and is easily capable of gaining a further 30kg on this lift, the best plan would be to steadily build a total across as many lifts as possible. After the bench press the first lifter would either need to be ahead by 30kg on the sub-total or, if both lifters have a relatively comparable bench press, it will be necessary to push the opponent to take risks on their deadlift. This can be achieved by the first lifter's coach registering for a weight heavier than they would be comfortable with and then reducing this before their turn, and any lot orders, come into play. This could force the opponent to increase their own opening deadlift and stay with it. Having been pushed to open higher, they may not fare well on subsequent attempts.

It is imperative for a coach to watch what other weights lifters are putting in for their second and third attempts, and it also helps to know their lifting history. For example, if there are three lifters all beginning within 5kg of your lifter's opening weight, it would be very useful to know if any of them are capable of making big incremental jumps. If so could they easily overtake your lifter. Similarly, it would be very useful to know if they are opening at a weight close to their limit, since this would indicate that they would have very little to add to the bar in subsequent attempts.

Tactics can make all the difference in the final round and may change almost up until the last minute since it is permissible to change the weight of the last attempt three times in total before actually performing the lift. To illustrate: lifter A may deadlift 145kg and then declare 150kg for their final attempt. However, they may change their mind and decide to go for a gold medal at 155kg so they change the attempt accordingly. Then lifter B puts in 155kg, so lifter A drops to 153kg in the hope that, by forcing B to declare the higher weight (thereby using their last change of weight), they may fail and A will win. Conversely, having the option to increase the next attempt after watching the opposition go first can be a tactical advantage.

The important thing is to observe other lifters closely and consider their body weight, their lot order, lifting sub-total and overall total that would be gained or not gained if the last lift was achieved or failed. This last-minute risk assess-ment and decision can make the difference between winning and losing.

The key to success in competition lies in understanding the opposition, the rules of the sport and combining excellent technique with strength under pressure to deliver the winning lift. The key point to remember in powerlifting is that it is the weights that are gained – and not lost – that matter: it is far better to gain 50kg than lose 65kg.

Types of Competition

Qualifying events
An event becomes a qualifying event (also known as a ranked event) when the national governing body and the corresponding international federation agree that the competition being held is a prerequisite for a particular championship. Qualifying standards will then apply and qualified referees should be in attendance at the event. For some events drug testing must be conducted and the lifters should be available for testing.

For example, the British championships are usually the prerequisite for the European championships, so if the lifter wishes to be considered for selection for the Europeans they must attend this championship. This would give the selectors the opportunity to observe them lift to the required standard. However, the qualifying total to be able to lift at a European championships could be achieved at designated ranked events across Great Britain prior to the British championships. It would be advisable for a lifter to lift in another ranked competition prior to the British championships so that if they had a bad performance at the British, other competition totals could be taken into account by the selection committee.

A non-qualification event may be refereed by lifters or divisional referees. At this level, manpower and facilities may be limited, there may be no kit checks and the organizers could be more relaxed on the timings between the weigh-in and actual lifting. For instance, weigh-in may take place the night before competition (although this is rare). All of this is fine as long as the lifters understand that no record attempts or lifting totals can be ratified by the Powerlifting Federations. Accepting this, these competitions do provide valuable opportunities for lifters to gain experience and measure their performance against others.

World championships

For all world championships (IPC and IPF) two athletes per body class per nation may compete, whereas in the Paralympics only one person per nation per body weight may complete in Paralympic (IPC) powerlifting.

WORLD CHAMPIONSHIPS (IPF AND IPC) VS PARALYMPICS POWERLIFTING (IPC ONLY)

IPF Powerlifting

- Not an Olympic sport.
- Built around the four-year World Championships cycle.

IPC Powerlifting

- Not an Olympic sport but a Paralympic sport (consisting solely of the bench press).
- Only one person per nation per body weight may complete in Paralympic (IPC) powerlifting.
- Training and events cycle follows the four-year Paralympic and Olympic cycle.

CHAPTER 10

DRUG TESTING

The sport of powerlifting works within the WADA (World Anti-Doping Association) guidelines, and all lifters selected to represent the Great Britain powerlifting teams should be prepared to take a drug test.

All UK sports that receive public funding are subject to drug testing. The majority of top lifters, world champions and record holders strongly advocate drug-free sport. Power-lifters frequently attend and deliver presentations in schools and clubs about the benefits of being healthy while competing in a drug free and fair sporting environment. Sir Chris Hoy, Dame Kelly Holmes and Baroness Tani Grey Thomson are just a few of Team GB's Olympic and Paralympic athletes who actively promote this via sporting programmes and advertising campaigns. One example is the UK Anti-Doping Federation's '100% me' campaign in which Team GB athletes publically state that all of their sporting performances were attributed to a 100 per cent natural effort. These individuals widely promote drug testing and argue for more stringent tests.

Athletes across all sports unite in the struggle to keep drug tests up-to-date and state-of-the-art, in order to catch cheats and deter athletes who may be considering taking drugs to enhance their sporting performance. This is a collaborative approach by top sports people and sporting organizations to encourage young aspiring champions to take a healthy approach to training and avoid the temptation of taking prohibited substances.

Out-of-Competition Drug Testing

Once a lifter has been able to string together some credible performances and is lifting successfully within the relevant qualifying totals for GB teams, they are likely to be selected for a British powerlifting squad. At this point they will be placed on the register for out-of-competition drug testing. This means that the testers can come to the lifter's home or place of training on any day of the year to conduct a test. The lifter will be required to keep one hour in every twenty-four free and let the anti-doping team know when this is and they must be prepared to be tested within that time slot. Most lifters pick a timeframe when they know they are always available, perhaps an hour before work. If, for some reason, they cannot be available at the time they have specified they may text, email or leave a voicemail with UK Anti-Doping to arrange another slot. They should also advise the federation if they are going to be away at a competition or on holiday so that appropriate arrangements can be made for testing to take place if required.

There is a three-strike rule: if a tester arrives at the place and time specified by the athlete and finds they are not there, and they are unable to contact and test them within the given hour, the athlete will receive a strike against their name. If a lifter receives three strikes they are liable to be banned from the sport for up to two years. In essence, avoiding a test equates to receiving a positive test result.

The athlete is responsible for the findings of their drug test, regardless of the result. Therefore, they must account for any substance that enters their body. This is a big responsibility that all athletes who wish to become true champions must accept.

Procedure for Recording Data

Fortunately, there is a comprehensive support network available to help lifters and coaches. As its name suggests, UK Anti-Doping is dedicated to protecting sport from the threat of doping in the UK. The organization has a comprehensive website which explains the benefits of staying free of banned substances, provides links to permitted medicines and substances and prohibited performance enhancing drugs, and clearly sets out the process for submitting samples for testing. It also provides downloadable factsheets for athletes, parents and coaches plus up-to-date posts, interactive blogs and information on the most recent global prohibited list.

If an athlete is unsure of any product, be it medication or supplement, they should check its name on the most up-to-date UK Anti-Doping website list (again, note it is the athlete's responsibility). This can be quickly done via mobile phone and internet connection. It is important to be very sure of the spelling and country of manufacture as the compounds and dosages may differ from country to country. It is worth noting that not all products are prohibited; most contraceptive pills are permitted, for example. Where substances are banned, there is nearly always an alternative to be found.

When an athlete identifies a clean substance that will serve their purpose on the UK Anti-Doping website, they should take screenshots of the date-stamped web pages where they found the information. This will enable them to prove, if required, that they had checked before taking the substance. They then need to check the batch number on every product they buy and consume and cross-reference it

against the listed substances. This is because the batch number on the tested product shown on the website might not be the same as on the purchased product. To help reduce this risk it is advisable for an athlete to purchase products via their individual Federation who will often have direct relationships with the manufacturing companies.

Medical Conditions

If medication needs to be prescribed by a doctor, a local general practitioner will be able to gain access to the correct lists. This way if the list changes between the time of the search and taking the drug, the lifter will have documented evidence to show that they took all precautionary steps.

A lifter's health is paramount and should never be compromised. There will be times when medication and banned drugs will need to be administered, for example following diagnosis of an ongoing illness such as diabetes, or post surgery. If an athlete becomes ill and requires medical attention they should seek the correct medical intervention. Structures and systems are in place to accommodate these situations.

Once an athlete is diagnosed with a legitimate medical condition, they must apply for a Therapeutic Use Exemption (TUE) which will allow them to use a prescribed prohibited substance or method to treat the condition. They will then be asked to see an independent doctor who will verify that they do indeed have the declared illness and that the prohibited substance is required for the athlete's health needs and serious risk may be incurred if the drug is not taken. The independent doctor will also check that there is no 'safe' alternative that could be used. Once satisfied that the necessary conditions have been met, they will then sign and timestamp the TUE application form. Athletes must ensure that the TUE is updated and keep it (or its reference number) with them so that they can fill in the data collection form when tested. Although the lifter's sample will show positive under analyses, it should match the information in the TUE, in which case the lifter will be granted a clear drug test.

Taking Supplements

The subject of supplements is a big area of contention within sport and powerlifting is no exception. Some say a good diet is all that is required. Others think it is near impossible to reach the top without supplements. Nevertheless, there is a huge market for these products. If using supplements, an athlete should learn to read and understand the terminology used on the container labels. This will help them to identify any banned substances.

If an athlete decides to use supplements they should be aware of the risk of product contamination during the manufacturing process. For example, they may be taking vitamin C and the company manufacturing it may also make a type of cough medicine that includes some banned ingredients. These may be distributed in the factory by a conveyer belt (or similar system) which is subsequently used to move the vitamin C. The vitamin C tablets can pick up trace elements of the banned substance and cause the athlete to test positive. It is the athlete's responsibility to research every substance they consume.

There are initiatives in place to help athletes navigate their way through this quagmire, one example being the Informed-Sport supplement testing and certification programme. All products bearing the Informed-Sport logo have been manufactured in facilities with high quality standards, have been tested for banned substances and are therefore safer for athletes to use.

Unfortunately this does not absolutely guarantee that there will be no contaminated products in circulation. All an athlete can do is follow strict evidence-based protocol and never take anything on face value. It should never be assumed that because one athlete seems to take a product and gain clear drug test results that other athletes will test clear too.

All athletes should be mindful of any products they purchase over the counter, whether at home or abroad, especially cold, flu and herbal remedies. As previously stated, preparations and compounds are likely to differ from country to country so the best option when travelling is for the athlete to take all their own medicines and supplements with the corresponding documentation.

The banned list may vary slightly from sport to sport. For instance, a snooker player would be under scrutiny if they took beta blockers since these help to block the effects of adrenaline, thereby relaxing the competitor. The player who is calm and has no excitable movements will be at an advantage. As such, beta blockers would be considered performance enhancers and a snooker player could be banned for taking them unless they could prove that they were needed for medical reasons and did not give them an advantage over other players.

A powerlifter would be at a disadvantage if they were too relaxed as they need to be in a heightened state of awareness. As such, they would find themselves under scrutiny if they appeared to be overdosing on caffeine as the resulting heighted state of awareness could be considered an advantage. A powerlifter could, therefore, be banned for extreme caffeine levels in their system although they are unlikely to be banned for taking beta blockers. Similarly, a snooker player is unlikely to be banned for taking caffeine.

All violations incur sanctions such as a ban from competing and/or a fine. If the offence is discovered at an international event the relevant lifting federation could also be fined. If the lifter is receiving government funding, any link with drugs in sport is likely to result in a loss of funding. Commercial funding may also be negatively impacted as sponsors may not wish to be associated with a lifter who is seen to be a cheat.

Coaches therefore have a great responsibility for educating, steering and directing their athletes to ensure they use the correct information and information sources. They too should maintain a clean and reputable attitude towards all prohibited substances in sport and adopt a zero tolerance approach. If a coach is found to be linked to any athlete taking drugs they too are likely to be fined and have their coaching licence revoked.

VIOLATIONS OF THE RULES LINKED WITH DRUGS IN SPORT

- Missing or refusing a drug test.
- Testing positive for banned substances.
- Tampering with and/or attempting to influence the testing procedure.
- Being in possession of any prohibited substances.
- Supplying and selling banned substances.

Testing Procedure

The athlete will be notified by the tester that they have been randomly selected to take a test. Once notified, the testing process has begun. If participating in a competition the athlete will report for testing at the venue and the tester will come to them (if at home they will carry out the test in the best available space). The athlete will be presented with several identical sealed collection vessels and must choose one. They will then provide a urine sample (with the tester witnessing the urine leaving the body) using the selected vessel. Having done so, they must choose a sampling bottle from a selection provided and transfer the sample into it as directed by the tester.

The validity of the sample depends on various factors. For example, it may be too strong due to dehydration from competing or there may not be enough of the sample to facilitate the full analysis required. If so, more will need to be given. Similarly, if the sample is shown to be the wrong consistency, for example if it has blood in it, a new sample will be required.

Once a valid sample has been collected certain information must be recorded and certified. This includes demographic data such as the athlete's age, sport and all the medication and supplements they have taken over the previous seven days. Any medication covered by a TUE must be recorded on the form. The athlete may state if they are unhappy with the way the procedure was carried out and include any other information they think may become relevant at a later date.

Increasingly, blood doping is being used as a test and is usually performed at top ranking events such as world championships. As the technology advances, this method is likely to be used more often.

The subject of prohibited substances and drug testing is complex and ever-changing and this chapter can only provide a snapshot of the current situation. Any UK lifter who is thinking of being placed on the drug testing register should contact their governing body and relevant UK sports agency, for example UK Sport. They must then commit to educating themselves on all aspects of drug testing, using correct and current information sources and terminology. Ignorance is no defence. They must also be prepared to follow the correct, evidence-based protocol by keeping a record of all medication and supplements taken, including dosages and time of consumption. As repeatedly stated the athlete is responsible at all times for everything that goes into their body. It is a huge responsibility and requires a 100 per cent commitment.

MINISTRY OF CULTURE G.S.S. - MINISTÈRE DE LA CULTURE S.G.S. OLYMPIC ATHLETIC CENTER OF ATHENS "SPIROS LOUIS" - CENTRE OLYMPIQUE ATHLÉTIQUE D' ATHÈNES "SPIROS LOUIS" DOPING CONTROL SERVICES - SERVICE DE CONTRÔLE DU DOPAGE	Form: Document:	EEN-120.01-EN DCM-120.01-F	EAOT EN ISO 9001:2000
	Page: Page:	Page 1/1: Page 1/1:	
DOPING CONTROL NOTIFICATION **NOTIFICATION DE CONTRÔLE DU DOPAGE**	Edition: Édition:	3.0	0399

Please print clearly with capital letters when filling in this form. / Veuillez remplir ce document en lettres majuscules.

Test Authorized by: Autorité ordonnante:	IPC	Venue-Location/Site:	INDOOR HALL OF KAVALA	Country-City: Pays-Cité:	GREECE - KAVALA
In competition: En compétition:	☒	Event: Événement:	8TH OPEN IPC POWERLIFTING EUROPEAN CHAMPIONSHIPS 2007
Out of competition: Hors compétition:	☐	Advance Notice: Notifié par advance:	☐	No Notice: Sans être notifié:	☐

Athlete's Information/Informations concernant le sportif:

Surname: Nom:		First Name: Prénom:	
Nationality: Nationalité:	GBR	Document Type and Number: Type et numéro de document:	LOT: No: 16
Gender: Male: ☒ Female: ☐ Sexe: Masculin: Féminin:		Sport/Discipline:	POWERLIFTING — 75 kg

Selection Criteria / Critères de sélection:	1ST PLACE	Biological Speciment Collected/Specimen Biologique prélevé:
		Urine: ☒ Urine EPO: ☐ Blood: ☐ Breath: ☐
		Urine: ☒ Urine EPO: ☐ Sang: ☐ Air expiré: ☐
Notification Time: Heure de Notification:	17 : 47	Date: Date:	13 / 06 / 20 07

You have been selected for doping control. You are required to report at the Doping Control Station with your Accreditation Pass (with photo) no later than ___ min after receipt of this notification. You will be chaperoned. You may also accompanied by one accredited representative. Failure to report for Doping Control within the given time limit and/or refusal to sign this form and/or refusal to provide a sample may constitute an anti-doping rule violation. By signing this Doping Control Notification you confirm that you have been notified of your selection and agree with all specified above.

Vous avez été désigné pour un contrôle du dopage. Vous devez vous présenter au poste de contrôle du dopage avec votre carte d' accréditation (avec photo), en ___ minutes au plus tard, du moment que vous aurez reçu cette notification. Vous serez toujours escorté. Vous pouvez vous faire accompagner d' un représentant accrédité. Votre non-présentation dans les délais impartis ou votre refus de signer ce document ou de fournir l' échantillon demandé pourra constituer une violation des régles antidopage. Votre signature a valeur d' accusé - réception de cette notification et confirme que vous étes d' accord avec ce qui a été dit ci-dessus.

| **Athlete's Signature/Signature du Sportif** | **Name & Signature of DC Escort:** **Nom & Signature de l' Escorte:** I hereby confirm that I have notified the athlete of his/her selection for doping control. Je confirme avoir notifié le sportif de sa sélection pour un contrôle du dopage. |

| Actual Reporting Time: S'est présenté au contrôle a: | : | Date: Date: | / / 20 |

The athlete arrived after the required reporting time . Le sportif est arrivé après les délais impartis.	☐	Without approval: Sans y avoir été autorisé:	☐	For valid reasons according to Article 5.4.5. for the International Standard for Testing: Pour des raisons valables Selon l' Article 5.4.5. des Standards Internationaux de Contrôle du Dopage :	☐
The athlete refused to sign the Notification: Le sportif a refusé de signer la Notification:	☐			The athlete failed to appear for doping control: Le sportif ne s'est pas présenté au contrôle du dopage:	☐
Name & Signature of DCO: Nom & Signature de l' ACD:					
Name & Signature of National/International Representative: Nom & Signature du Représentant National/International:				Absent: Absent:	☐

WHITE CORY: Doping Control Services/OAKA **PINKCOPY:** Ordering Authority **YELLOW COPY:** Athlete
FEUILLET BLANC: Service de contrôle du dopage/ OAKA **FEUILLET ROSE:** Autorité ordonnante **FEUILLET JAUNE:** Sportif

Doping Control Notification form.

GLOSSARY

1RM (One Repetition Maximum)   One repetition lifted with maximum load (weight).

A and B groups   A process that divides athletes into the groups in which they will lift during a competition.
adaptation   When the body and mind adjust to accommodate increased tonnage lifted.
add-on for amputee   The amount of weight, in kilos, which is added to the lifter's body weight in lieu of the missing limb.
alternating grip   A lifting grip, associated with the deadlift, where one hand has the palm facing toward the body and the other facing away from the body.
analysis   The process of breaking a complex topic or substance into smaller parts to gain a better understanding of it.
anatomy   The science discipline concerned with the bodily structure of human beings.
anterior muscle chain   A group of muscles, tendons and ligaments located at the front of the body, including for example the quadriceps and the chest.
anti doping   The underlying concept and organizations working to keep sport free from inhibited performance-enhancing drugs.
arch   Bench press body posture, designed to reduce the distance the bar has to travel.
athlete   A person who demonstrates the genetic propensity or the acquired traits such as strength, agility and endurance that are required in sport, especially those performed in competitive contexts.
athlete-specific   Describes a process that places the athlete, their needs and subsequent perform-ance at its core.
athlete service agreement   Agreed engagement between athlete and the funding authority.

bar   Competition powerlifting bar which is designed to hold in excess of 400kg for the express purpose of enabling lifters to lift huge tonnage (weights).
bench press   Known as the key exercise which demonstrates upper body strength, in which the athlete lies face up on a bench and the bar is held at arm's length; once under control the bar is lowered down to the chest, held momentarily, then pushed back up to the starting position.
bioimpedance   The response of a living organism to an externally applied electric current, which is a non-invasive method to measure blood flow and body composition.
biomechanics   The science of the forces exerted by muscles and gravity on the skeletal structure.
bomb out   To fail to gain a successful lift in one category (squat bench or deadlift) and consequently no longer be in the competition.
box squat   A back squat where the athlete descends to and momentarily rests on a strategically placed bench/box at the bottom of the squat, after which they return to the standing position.
BPA   British Paralympics Association.

classification   A system based on the medical model of disability which divides athletes into groups or sports by the nature of their impairment and direct function of each of their limbs.

coach   An individual who empowers athletes to achieve their potential by undertaking different roles, such as tutor, educator or trainer, as the situation requires.

code of conduct   A list of behaviours expected when representing a team or country such as Team GB.

code of ethics   A guide of principles designed to help professionals conduct business honestly and with integrity.

collars   Safety devices to secure weights to the bar.

core   Basic muscles concentrated in the centre of the body, including the abdominals and back muscles, which control balance, total body support and alignment.

cycle   A period of training.

development   An athlete's improvement which indicates their potential to gain medals; this is directly linked to the level of attainment required to be eligible to be invited onto a world-class funded sporting programme.

deadlift   Known as a true test of back strength, in which the lifter bends down to the bar, which is placed on the floor parallel to their feet, grips it tightly and pulls the weight up, primarily by pushing through their feet and pulling up through their hands, and leading up to standing erect with the weight in the hands.

de load   A measured period of time when the training load is reduced, often by lifting less weight and conducting more repetitions during training sessions.

discs   Round weights, identified by numbers in kilos written on each side, which are loaded onto the powerlifting bar.

exercise   Structured and repetitive bodily movements that individuals undertake in order to improve or maintain fitness and/or health.

fast bench   A lift comprised of the same movement as the bench press with faster speed during the accent phase (see bench press).

flat back   Neutral position of the spine when lying prone and face up on a bench.

flexor   A muscle, when contracted, that bends a limb or other part of the body.

focus   The ability to concentrate and narrow your attention effectively to a particular situation or element within a situation, and not be distracted by outside influences.

form   The correct body posture and body shape to be held when performing a lift.

gluteus maximus   The largest muscles that make up the buttocks.

gluteus medius   The middle size muscles that make up the buttocks.

gluteus minimus   The smaller size muscles which make up the buttocks.

goal setting   An academic theory that suggests that people are motivated by clear, specific, incremental targets, as opposed to generic requests or thoughts.

grip   The position of the hand on the bar in any given lift.

high performance   Sporting performance outcomes that yield a medal at a world championships or Olympics and Paralympics.

IPC   International Paralympics powerlifting Committee.

IPF   International Powerlifting Federation.

incline dumb bell press   A bench press movement conducted in a sitting incline position with a dumbbell in each hand, to train the pectoralis major (primarily upper portion), triceps, and anterior deltoid muscles.

inhibited substance (steroid)   An artificial hormone that enables the human body to recover far more quickly and promotes excelled muscle growth and adaptation, but which in the context of sport is banned.

intensity   The average force and power that the athlete works at during a training session and/or per block of training. To ascertain average intensity divide the training session's tonnage lifted by the number of repetitions completed (this formula can also be employed for the intensity of each individual lift or exercise).

kinesiology   The science of the mechanics of body movements.

lat pull down   Machine exercise aimed to target the latissimus dorsi (lats) upper back, to train the latissimus dorsi, teres major, trapezius (lower portion), rhomboids and biceps (see Chapter 1).

levers   In performing a lift, where one limb is longer than another the muscles and bones work together as a series of levers, creating an axis.

lifting suit   A garment designed to support the body/torso hips whilst performing a lift.

loader   A trained individual who specializes in the order of lifting and how to place the correct denomination of weights onto a powerlifting bar. They are experts in shadowing a lifter when performing exercises with heavy weights, and they have a full understanding of the safety issues within powerlifting and know at which points to intervene to keep the lifter safe.

lot order   The number assigned to a lifter during a competition which depicts who should go first for the weigh in, and if two lifters wish to attempt to lift the same weight; to ensure fair play the numbers are obtained through a random number generator.

mental imagery   Visual and other information that is not currently being perceived by the sense organs but is simulated in the mind, providing the opportunity for mental rehearsal of an event or competition.

motivation   Factors that initiate, steer and/or maintain behaviour.

PB (Personal Best)   The best performance of a lift or exercise.

pectorals   Major and minor chest muscles.

performance curves   A graph which plots the progress of an athlete's performance in relation to pre-set sporting targets.

performance goals   Behavioural outcomes or targets achieved by an athlete.

performance marker   Performance measures for prediction and evaluation.

platform   The official designated area for competitive lifting.

posterior muscle chain   A group of muscles, tendons and ligaments located at the back of the body, for example the gluteus.

pre-hab (pre-habilitation)   A group of exercises to strengthen weak points to prevent injury occurring, designed and led by a physiotherapist in conjunction with the coach.

pressing (*see* **pushing**)

GLOSSARY

prone rows   Exercises performed while lying in a horizontal position to enable the development of the back and shoulders; often performed with dumbbells but can be done with resistance bands and/or powerlifting bar.
psychological skills   Cognitive strategies devised to enhance performance in sport.
pulling   Pulling the weight away from the floor.
pushing   Pushing the weight away from the body.

quad leg extension   Machine exercise designed to train the quadriceps muscles: rectis femoris, vastus lateralis, vastus medialis and vastus intermedius.

rep (repetition)   One full movement of an exercise.
re-hab (rehabilitation)   Therapy directed towards improving body function that has been lost or diminished by injury or disease.
round system (rising bar)   During the competition the bar is progressively loaded to heavier weights as each attempt is made; it is only reduced once the round has finished.

secondary exercises (assistance)   Resistance exercises which are not one of the three powerlifting lifts.
scapula   Shoulder blade.
set   A selected number of repetitions performed as a group.
sporting injury   Any physical or medical condition that prevents an athlete from participating in a training session or competition, broadly classified as either traumatic or overuse injury, and ranging from back misalignment to muscle and ligament sprains.
squat   Known as the king of leg exercises, strengthening the legs and back, in which the athlete stands with the weight and powerlifting bar sitting across their shoulders with their hands gripping the bar; once they have the weight under control they descend with the weight until their hips reach just below the knees, and then ascend back to the original standing position.
stability under load   Achieved when a lifter is able to control the powerlifting bar and prevent it and their limbs from being pulled out of line or toppling over.
sticking point   A point during a lift at which the lifter encounters a stronger resistance, and the tempo of the bar slows down dramatically and can even stop.
strength   A term used in powerlifting for the demonstration of force when producing a one-repetition maximum lift.
strength to body weight ratio   The amount of weight lifted compared to the actual weight of the person lifting the weight; the person who lifts the most weight compared to their own body weight is considered to be the strongest.
subcutaneous fat layer   The fatty or adipose tissue which sits directly under the skin layers.
supplements   Minerals, vitamins and other related products designed and used to support the nutritional content of the diet.

Talent ID (Talent Identification)   Multi-disciplinary screening of athletes to identify those with potential; each sport has its own qualifying totals and requirements which when achieved represent talent that is thought to produce top class athletes.
technical meeting   A meeting held prior a competition, designed to ensure that all concerned are informed of pending schedules, that the rules of the sport are upheld and fair play is adhered to at all times.

thorax   The area in the upper body between the neck and the diaphragm, partially encased by the ribs and containing the heart and lungs; in general, the chest.

tonnage   The sum total of the kilograms lifted in a training session multiplied by the number of repetitions for each set completed during the session.

torque force   A force to rotate an object about an axis fulcrum or pivot; just as a force is a push or a pull, a torque can be thought of as a twist to an object. In this context, the force to move a weight with the body acting as the axis, for example knee torque.

total   The amount of kilograms lifted across all successful attempts in competition.

training programme   Detailed schedules/plans created towards obtaining specific lifting targets or competition outcomes.

TUE (Therapeutic Use Exemption)   Process whereby an appointed medical doctor validates medication that is on the prohibited list for an athlete with a validated reason for taking it.

UKAD   United Kingdom Anti Doping in sport.

volume   The quantity of the work undertaken in a training session, which may be expressed in terms of the number of lifts and or completed individual exercises.

WADA   World Anti Doping Association

weight class   Standardized weight classification system that decides who lifts against who.

wrist knee wrap   A woven fabric that when applied around the knee or wrist provides adding security against the torque force and pull from the weight being lifted.

World Class Performance Programme   A British funded programme designed to offer athletes with potential to represent the UK and gain a medal at world championships and above, governed by government and sporting agencies such as the Olympic association, and offering a full network of support and related services.

world ranking list   The list of the athletes ratified lifting totals across the comparator group.

FURTHER READING

Acknowledgement

In preparing this book the author has drawn on the ethos of the following agencies and governing bodies.

References

Morgan, A.P., Sport and Exercise Psychology (Routledge, 2004)
Lear, J., Skilful Weightlifting (A&C Black, 1991)

Useful Contacts

British Weightlifting Association (covers IPC Powerlifting and British Weightlifting), www.britishweightlifting.org.
English Federation of Disability Sport, www.efds.co.uk.
English Institute of Sport, www.eis2win.co.uk.
European Powerlifting Federation, www.europowerlifting.org.
Great Britain Powerlifting Federation (GBPF), www.gbpf.org/uk.
International Paralympic Committee (IPC), www.paralympic.org/Powerlifting.
International Powerlifting Federation (IPF), www.powerlifting-ipf.com.
Scottish Institute of Sport, www.sisport.com.
Sports Coach UK, www.sportscoachuk.org.
Sport England, www.sportengland.org.
International Coaching Federation UK, www.coachfederation.org.uk.
UK Anti-Doping, www.ukad.org.uk.
UK Sport, www.uksport.gov.uk.
World Anti Doping Agency (WADA), www.wada-ama.org.
Welsh Institute of Sport, www.sportwales.org.uk.
Women's Sports Foundation, www.womenssportsfoundation.org.

INDEX

INDEX